THE JOHNS HOPKINS GUIDE *TO*
EVERYDAY
PSYCHOLOGICAL FIRST AID

A JOHNS HOPKINS HEALTH PRESS BOOK

THE JOHNS HOPKINS GUIDE *TO*

EVERYDAY PSYCHOLOGICAL FIRST AID

A Practical Approach to Helping Family, Friends,
Coworkers, and Others Cope

GEORGE S. EVERLY, JR. & JEFFREY M. LATING

JOHNS HOPKINS UNIVERSITY PRESS
Baltimore

© 2026 Johns Hopkins University Press
All rights reserved. Published 2026
Printed in the United States of America on acid-free paper

2 4 6 8 9 7 5 3 1

Johns Hopkins University Press
2715 North Charles Street
Baltimore, Maryland 21218
www.press.jhu.edu

Library of Congress Cataloging-in-Publication Data is available.

ISBN 978-1-4214-5382-8 (hardcover)
ISBN 978-1-4214-5383-5 (paperback)
ISBN 978-1-4214-5384-2 (ebook)

A catalog record for this book is available from the British Library.

Special discounts are available for bulk purchases of this book.
For more information, please contact Special Sales at
specialsales@jh.edu.

EU GPSR Authorized Representative
LOGOS EUROPE, 9 rue Nicolas Poussin,
17000, La Rochelle, France
E-mail: Contact@logoseurope.eu

CONTENTS

TEN   160
Panic

ELEVEN   174
Traumatic Stress

TWELVE   189
Eating Disorders

PART I
READ THIS SECTION FIRST

FOUNDATIONS OF PSYCHOLOGICAL FIRST AID (PFA)

Welcome to *The Johns Hopkins Guide to Everyday Psychological First Aid (E-PFA): A Practical Approach to Helping Family, Friends, Coworkers, and Others Cope*

It's probably obvious, but we will say it anyway. In every home and business there should be a physical first aid kit that includes a basic instruction manual. Why? To paraphrase John Lennon, because "life happens when you're busy making other plans." A physical first aid manual provides guidance on how you can respond to acute physical injuries, among other things. Even though it doesn't teach the practice of medicine or surgery, this type of manual can be very useful — perhaps even lifesaving.

It's probably less obvious, so we need to say it. We believe every home and business should have a psychological first aid manual that provides guidance on how you might respond to acute psychological injuries. Why? That's right, because "life happens when you're busy making other plans." As you might guess, the purpose of this manual is to provide such guidance. Psychological injuries (or acute psychological distress) include things like anxiety, grief, guilt, and even reactive depression. Even though psychological first aid (PFA) is not counseling or psychotherapy, it can still be very useful.

This manual utilizes a standardized five-step model as a general guide. As a foundation, we provide background material on the nature and prevalence of certain forms of psychological distress. In addition, we provide examples of and tactical options for how someone might activate the model for each type. Last, we provide examples of dialogue—what the person attempting to help might say. The mechanisms of activation and the example dialogues are just that—examples. They are not intended to be used verbatim. No two interventions will be exactly alike. This is because each intervention must be tailored to the specific needs of the unique person and their unique situation.

This manual is an extension of our previous text, *The Johns Hopkins Guide to Psychological First Aid*. That book and the research it is based on were designed to assist emergency services, health care professionals, the military, and disaster responders as they aid survivors (and themselves) during and after adversity, trauma, and disaster. Compiling it was a journey we began in the late 1980s, one that has taken us to the burning oil fields of Kuwait after the first Gulf War, the rubble piles of Ground Zero in New York City after the terrorist attacks of September 11, 2001, war zones in Eastern Europe, the impact zones of three pandemics (Hong Kong, Singapore, and the United States), and countless hurricanes, floods, and fires in over 30 countries on 6 continents. Acknowledging that stress, depression, guilt, and even trauma are not restricted to first responders and the military, and furthermore, acknowledging the importance of psychological health for all people in all aspects of daily living, we created this manual of everyday psychological first aid (E-PFA)—a simple, step-by-step approach to helping friends, family, coworkers, and others cope.

This is not a clinical textbook. It is not a guide to the diagnosis and treatment of psychiatric emergencies. And it is certainly not intended to replace professional psychological or psychiatric care. Rather, it is a set of evidence-informed and evidenced-based options for assisting someone in distress. The examples included in this manual largely consist of educational, cathartic, cognitive, and behavioral stress management interventions, not therapy interventions. Helping people in acute distress often consists of helping them feel empowered. All these techniques can do just that. The English philosopher, statesman, and scientist Sir Francis Bacon believed that information and education equaled power. Psychologists have long known the value of letting people vent, a process known as catharsis. Cognitive strategies, which help individuals regulate their thoughts and emotions, were first developed by the ancient Greek philosophers as viewpoints from which to live one's life. These same principles were adapted by modern psychologists as guidance for everyday living. For example, stress management techniques have been the focus of self-help books for over 100 years.

The step-by-step checklists included in the applied chapters are potential starting places for providing assistance. Once again, they are not scripts to be read or employed verbatim. They are merely examples of how the everyday psychological first aid model we have developed might be applied and what the interventions might sound like. It is important to reiterate that PFA interventions must be tailored to the unique person and their unique situation. That said, to help someone in emotional distress, we no longer have to rely on a compassionate heart or a verbal "Hail

Mary" alone. E-PFA provides a structure for helping people cope. And you never know when you may use it. As Winston Churchill once noted, "To each there comes in their lifetime a special moment when they are figuratively tapped on the shoulder and offered the chance to do a very special thing. . . . What a tragedy if that moment finds them unprepared or unqualified for that which could have been their finest hour."

The manual is divided into two parts:

Part One, "Foundations of Psychological First Aid," lays the essential groundwork for understanding and applying PFA.
Part Two, "Everyday Psychological First Aid for Common Psychological Injuries and Crises," offers specific, practical guidelines on how to use E-PFA for a wide variety of psychological injuries.

Most chapters in Part Two are relatively short since we use outlines, bullet points, and checklists as often as possible. A few chapters are necessarily longer, such as "Intoxication" (Chapter Thirteen), to cover a wide array of variations on the core theme. Each chapter in Part Two follows the same basic structure: scenario exemplifying the condition; definition of the condition; key features of the condition; potential E-PFA recommendations; and a sample dialogue. While some of the dialogues may sound somewhat inflexible, it's again important to note that they were not written to be applied verbatim and do not rely solely on everyday language. This is because their application will vary greatly across settings and individuals.

As helpful as we believe this manual can be, it is no substitute for professional mental health assessment or treatment. Whenever you are in doubt about how to assist another person in distress, consider reaching out to mental health professionals or even calling 9-1-1 (local emergency services) or 9-8-8 (Suicide and Crisis Lifeline).

ONE | What Is Psychological First Aid?

YOU ARE IN THE MIDDLE seat on a five-hour nonstop flight. After about an hour you notice that the young man sitting next to you in the window seat, whom you do not know, is shaking and lightly perspiring. You ask if he is okay. He responds he has a fear of flying and is experiencing a panic attack. What do you do?

You are a passenger in a car driven by a close friend. While in heavy traffic, another car cuts you off. Your friend experiences road rage. He yells at the other driver, blows the horn, and starts tailgating. What do you do?

Your 16-year-old daughter comes to you with tears in her eyes. Her boyfriend of eight months has just ended their relationship. He had been dating another person, unbeknownst to your daughter, and finally broke up with her to be with the other person. This was your daughter's first serious relationship. What do you say?

You attend the funeral of the daughter of one of your best friends. She died in a tragic auto accident at age 18. After the funeral, you and about 30 other people go to your friend's home. You see your friend alone, crying. You approach him to ask if there is anything you can do. He says, "Why did this happen? It's not fair. She had her whole life in front of her. It's my fault. I should have seen it coming?" What do you say?

These scenarios, which you'll encounter in modified form again later in the manual, have two things in common. First, they show people in acute psychological distress. Second, they illustrate where psychological first aid (PFA) could be used to reduce that distress.

Most, if not all, readers of this manual have witnessed another person in distress. Perhaps it was an acute physical crisis, like an accident or a sudden illness. At that moment you probably wished that you were skilled in physical first aid. But sometimes it was an emotional crisis: another person seemed anxious, fearful, depressed, or just overwhelmed. Regardless of whether it was a friend, a family member, a coworker, or even a stranger, in that situation you were likely motivated to offer some form of support to ease their distress. Sometimes your best efforts are effective, but sometimes they are not. Sometimes, despite your best efforts, your actions appear to make matters worse, seeming to intensify the other person's distress. At such times perhaps you lamented the absence of a psychological magic bullet that would immediately end their suffering and lead them to realize the promise you might have made that "Everything will be okay."

Sadly, however, there is no such magic bullet, no verbal "Hail Mary." Still, over the last 100 years a concept and approach have evolved to help ease emotional distress and suffering. This approach is called psychological first aid (PFA). Just as you can learn physical first aid, virtually any adult can learn PFA. In fact, research dating back decades has shown that you do not need a degree in psychology or mental health to be effective in helping another person reduce acute distress (Durlak, 1979; Eisdorpher & Golann, 1969; Everly & Lating, 2022).

Psychological First Aid Defined

The best way to conceptualize PFA, as we use the term, is as the psychological analogue to physical first aid. PFA is a form of psychological crisis intervention. More specifically, PFA can be simply defined as a supportive and compassionate presence designed to:

1) stabilize acute psychological distress (prevent the stress from getting worse);
2) reduce acute psychological distress (reduce the intensity of the stress);
3) promote resilience (foster the ability to bounce back); and/or
4) facilitate access to continued or more advanced assistance, if needed.

At the core of PFA is human connection, communication, and interpersonal support. Oprah Winfrey once asserted, "Great communication begins with connection." According to American author and entrepreneur John Rohn, "If you just communicate, you can get by. But if you communicate skillfully, you can work miracles." PFA is artfully applying the science of skillful and supportive communications in a compassionate manner. PFA does not entail diagnosing, nor does it entail treatment in the traditional psychotherapeutic sense. It's simply a psychological Band-Aid— but one so important that even the editors of a prestigious science magazine declared that everyone should learn to apply it. Our opinion, and the foundation of this manual, is that anyone who can learn to apply physical first aid should learn PFA.

Why Is Psychological First Aid Important?

Have you noticed that stress is everywhere? Generally speaking, life can be challenging. And sometimes, through no fault of their own, people find themselves in the wrong place at the wrong time, triggering stress that becomes disorienting, disabling, and perhaps even catastrophic. But nature has provided human beings with the ability to protect themselves against and even bounce back from disabling stress if it does occur. Research tells us that psychological connection and support from others is a powerful predictor of human health and the single best predictor of resilience (Ozer et al., 2003). So important is human connection that the inclination to form relationships with others is biologically hardwired. On the other hand, not only does the absence of support leave a person with less interpersonal capital to draw on during highly stressful times, but it is associated with health problems such as depression, substance misuse, and even premature death. Here's the good news: PFA not only fuels connection; it also offers a quick and effective way to provide interpersonal support and foster resilience when most needed. PFA can be applied to a wide range of psychological injuries, distress, and dysphoria.

It's been said we live in an age of anxiety. Anxiety can be thought of as apprehension and increased stress arousal. Uncertainty resides at the center of anxiety. Most people dread uncertainty. So important is the need for certainty that Virginia Satir, a pioneering author and an instrumental developer of family systems therapy, noted, "People prefer the certainty of misery to the misery of uncertainty." Human connection and interpersonal support presented in a PFA framework combat anxiety. In some instances, it can combat uncertainty by providing constructive information about what to expect, how to cope, or even how to problem-solve. It can provide reassurance and normalization so that people do not feel they are the only ones to experience distress. At the very least, PFA-based interpersonal connection can offer a caring presence that allows a person in distress to vent their anxiety, fears, grief, frustrations, disappointments, and anger.

No man is an island,
entire of itself . . .
Any man's death diminishes me,
because I am involved
in mankind; and therefore
never send to know
for whom the bell tolls;
it tolls for thee.

John Donne (1572–1631), Meditation XVII, 1624

The notion captured by English poet, scholar, and cleric John Donne has rung true through the ages, yet loneliness plagues society. Loneliness is a condition characterized by being detached, being prone to melancholy, and having few meaningful interpersonal connections. Loneliness has been shown to increase the risk of early death by 32% (Holt-Lunstad et al., 2015). Loneliness is not only a major cause of depression; it is associated with anxiety, sleep disturbance, alcohol misuse, and even suicidal thoughts. In 2023, the US Surgeon General called loneliness an "epidemic." A survey conducted by the American Psychiatric Association in 2024 found that 30% of adults had experienced feelings of loneliness at least once a week over the preceding year, while 10% said they were lonely "every day." A YouGov survey (Ballard, 2019) found that 22% of millennials indicated they have no friends.

While PFA is not a cure for loneliness, it can often be the first step toward recognition of the problem and serve as a catalyst for addressing the epidemic of loneliness. It can be a powerful way to communicate caring while underscoring the value of every human life. Loneliness has been enshrined in innumerable songs, such as "One" written by Harry Nilsson and performed by the rock group Three Dog Night. The song is best known for its opening line about "one" being the loneliest number, which is likely not merely a catchy phrase but maybe also Nilsson's commentary on society in the late 1960s. He then writes about how the word "no" is a sad experience that possibly carries the weight of loneliness. Before that, Bobby Vinton wrote and performed the song "Mr. Lonely" in 1964.

Loneliness is not simply an empty feeling; it can lead to catastrophe. In 2022, over 49,000 people in the US died by suicide (Centers for Disease Control and Prevention, 2024). Suicide is not an isolated action; it often represents a culmination of intolerable desperation. There are many paths that can lead to suicidal thoughts or action, and PFA may prevent them from leading to tragedy.

The Golden Gate Bridge in San Francisco, which opened on May 27, 1937, is one of the world's most famous structures, known for its beauty and architecture. But it is also known as a place where people go to attempt suicide. Over 1,800 people are believed to have jumped from the bridge since its completion, with only 39 known survivors. One of the most compelling stories of those who survived is that of Kevin Hines. On September 25, 2000, at age 19, Hines let go of the bridge's protective railing and fell more than 200 feet, hitting the water at a speed of 75 miles per hour. The fall only took four seconds, but the instant Hines was in the air he knew he did not want to die. "I realized I made the greatest mistake of my life," he later recalled (Health Central, 2024). After surviving the fall, he became afraid he was going to drown. But that was not to be. A sea lion kept pushing him to the surface until the Coast Guard rescued him. Today, Hines is a leading international advocate of suicide prevention with award-winning books and films to his credit.

What does the story of Kevin Hines have to do with PFA? Of the 39 people who have survived a fall from the Golden Gate Bridge, 20 admitted to instantly regretting their actions. But more significantly, Hines said it was the belief that no one cared that fueled his suicidal intention.

According to Hines, a suicidal person "needs to hear what I needed to hear. That we care about you, your life does matter, and that all we want is for you to stay" and "If someone had looked at me on that bridge or on that bus and said that to me, I would have begged for help" (Health Central, 2024).

Someone trained in PFA could have been that voice. PFA might have prevented Hines's jump. It can be the voice of caring that prevents needless deaths from suicide every year.

History of Psychological First Aid

Offering a compassionate and supportive presence based on effective communication lies at the foundation of PFA. This notion dates back over 2,000 years. Somewhere around 70 BC, Roman statesman Marcus Tullius Cicero is reported to have said that friends multiply happiness and divide sadness — or it might have been Linus speaking to a forlorn Charlie Brown, but you get the point. "With a Little Help from My Friends" is a song written by John Lennon and Paul McCartney of the Beatles, released in 1967 on the album *Sgt. Pepper's Lonely Hearts Club Band*. Its refrain emphasizes how we all rely on friends to get by.

Yes, we do feel empowered when someone has our back. And yes, we do try harder with a little help from our friends. Friends are those who rush to help when others are rushing away. But you do not have to be a "friend" to help someone in distress; you do, however, need more than good intentions. You need skill in compassionate, targeted communications and support.

The formal foundations of the science of PFA can be traced back to the two world wars, which began in 1914 and 1939. Traditional psychiatric treatments for stress and trauma were not effective at fostering resilience among military members. In contrast, principles of acute psychological crisis intervention—such as normalizing stress reactions, offering reassurance, and promoting camaraderie—more than tripled rates of resilience. During World War II, the US Merchant Marine even developed a PFA curriculum for its crews.

During the Cold War, the American Psychiatric Association (APA) recommended PFA training for Civil Defense workers and other first responders (APA, 1954), emphasizing that, as noted above, support from others is the single best predictor of human resilience (Ozer et al., 2003). In the wake of the terrorist attacks and World Trade Center disaster of September 11, 2001, the Institute of Medicine (2003) wrote, "There has been a growing movement in the world to develop a concept similar to physical first aid for coping with stressful and traumatic events in life. This strategy has been known by a number of names but is most commonly referred to as psychological first aid (PFA)" (p. 4).

More recently, and in response to the impact of the COVID-19 pandemic, the editors of the highly regarded magazine *Scientific American* noted, "All of us need to sustain and enhance our psychological resilience to weather the daily toll of activity restrictions, rising case numbers, hospitalizations and deaths. A set of simple measures known as psychological first aid or mental health first aid can enable people to help family, friends and others in their communities" (Editors, 2021, p. 10).

Perhaps as a testament to the perceived value of PFA, a free online class teaching the evidence-based model, developed in conjunction with the Johns Hopkins Center for Public Health Preparedness and published on the learning platform Coursera, has had over 590,000 people sign up worldwide. Not surprisingly, the editors of *Scientific American* asserted, "Everyone should take it."

Caution

We've reviewed the importance of interpersonal support, its history, and its apparent simplicity. But assisting someone in acute distress is not as easy as it may appear. No matter how good our intentions, whenever we dare to enter a person's experience of distress or injury, there are risks. We could inadvertently delay or divert the person from getting more appropriate or intense assistance. Or in trying to reassure them, we might inadvertently seem dismissive of genuinely serious concerns. Or, conversely, we might overreact to what is actually an acute, short-lived, "normal" stress reaction. We might become enmeshed in the situation, adding unneeded complexity and stress for ourselves. In myriad ways, we could make things considerably worse.

The latter possibility was recognized by the eighth-century BC Greek poet Homer who, in *The Iliad*, described a mother's failed attempt to aid her son. Upon learning of the death of his best friend in battle, the warrior Achilles descended into vengeful rage. As most parents can relate, his mother, Thetis, tried to comfort him—but more importantly to dissuade him from seeking vengeance, knowing it would have a tragic ending. She failed to calm him. Ignoring her advice, Achilles acted on his rage and died in battle—as she had predicted.

How many times have you tried to warn someone of an adverse outcome, and how many times have you been ignored or placated? The risk of making things worse despite sincere efforts was perhaps best captured in writing in 1855, when Henry Bohn included the saying "The road to hell is paved with good intentions" in *A*

Hand-book of Proverbs. It is a phrase with versions dating back to the 1600s.

The core principles of PFA have been taught to law enforcement, emergency medical technicians, clergy, teachers, university administrators, hostage negotiators, air traffic controllers, clinicians in emergency departments, flight crews of airlines, security guards, paramedics, and even frontline managers in business and industry (being a supervisor sometimes requires being a confidant). The importance of recognizing and attending to psychological dynamics at the workplace gained prominence with Douglas McGregor's classic book, *The Human Side of Enterprise* (McGregor, 1960). Today its relevance is reflected in a 2022 survey, which found that Gen Z (born in 1996 or later) expect their supervisors to be not only technically supportive but also psychologically supportive (Deloitte Global, 2022). Proper training in and implementation of the principles of PFA can advance this goal. It is worth repeating a quote from Winston Churchill, first mentioned in the introduction to Part One, that captures the essence of the importance of learning PFA: "To each there comes in their lifetime a special moment when they are figuratively tapped on the shoulder and offered the chance to do a very special thing, unique to them and fitted to their talents. What a tragedy if that moment finds them unprepared or unqualified for that which could have been their finest hour."

The Johns Hopkins Model of Everyday Psychological First Aid (E-PFA)

This manual is intended for use in the household, the workplace, and beyond. It offers a streamlined, practical expansion of the PFA approach presented in the online Coursera course and detailed in the clinical textbook *The Johns Hopkins Guide to Psychological First*

Aid (Everly & Lating, 2022). The focus here is on addressing acute psychological injuries, distress, and dysphoria triggered by a range of stressors, including daily conflicts and frustrations, economic worries, developmental crises (especially relevant for adolescents), relationship discord, substance use, loss and grief, fear, and both direct and vicarious traumas. It offers ways that everyday psychological first aid (E-PFA) can be used to mitigate their impact. The model presented is a straightforward, practical approach to PFA that can be used by just about any adult, anywhere. As noted in the introduction to this book, the model of PFA presented in this manual is a simplified variation of the RAPID-PFA model published in the clinical textbook *The Johns Hopkins Guide to Psychological First Aid* (Everly and Lating, 2022), which we have adapted here for the household, workplace, and beyond.

The core elements of PFA have been validated with individuals (Everly et al., 2016), groups (Despeaux et al., 2019), and communities (McCabe, Everly, et al., 2014 McCabe, Semon, et al., 2014). They will be described in more detail in Chapters Two and Three. We believe that PFA can be effectively taught beginning in young adulthood (Durlak, 1979; Eisdorpher & Golann, 1969; Jacobs, 2016; SAMHSA, 2015), and that a degree in psychology or mental health is not required to learn it (Everly et al., 2012; Everly & Kennedy, 2019; Everly et al., 2014). While the principles of PFA can be introduced earlier, we are concerned about the potential emotional costs for younger people, given their relative lack of life experience and ongoing expressive development. Accordingly, this manual is designed primarily for use by adults over age 21.

Our nonclinical, simplified, adaptation of the RAPID-PFA model, which we refer to from this point forward as everyday psychological first aid (E-PFA), consists of an easy-to-use checklist-based formula. The effectiveness of the model may reside in its simplicity. At its core, E-PFA consists of five steps, summarized in Table 1.1.

Table 1.1
Everyday Psychological First Aid (E-PFA)

---

1) Introduce yourself, offer to help, and set expectations, as appropriate. Help de-escalate stress if necessary.
2) Gather information.
3) Clarify and distill the main points you've heard.
4) Provide assistance.
5) Make a plan. Follow up.

In the chapters that follow in Part One, we will expand on each of the five steps. In Part Two, we will show how the model can be applied to everyday life and to psychological injuries of various types and intensity as they may arise in households, workplaces, and communities.

KEY POINTS

1) Simple, easy to use, and practical—these are the keys to effective utilization of E-PFA. The checklist approach used throughout this manual is designed to support that goal. Checklists have been shown to improve effectiveness of tasks in health care, including surgical safety, medication understanding, and accomplishing daily goals (Pronovost et al., 2003; Winters et al., 2009). To enhance ease and practicality, this manual will use enumerated lists and bullet-point checklists whenever possible.

2) It is generally recommended that every household have a handbook on physical first aid, a tool whose use can reduce physical pain and suffering, and in some cases even save lives. Just as physical injuries occur, psychological "injuries" can occur as well. So shouldn't you have a practical guide to psychological first aid? Now you can. When prudently applied, the guidelines in this manual can reduce psychological pain and suffering, and perhaps even save a life.

3) The everyday psychological first aid (E-PFA) model is derived from the evidence-based Johns Hopkins RAPID-PFA model, originally developed for public health emergencies and disasters. E-PFA is designed for everyday use—with friends, family, coworkers, and others—during times of crisis or acute distress, including situations where someone is unable to function effectively.

4) E-PFA may be thought of as a psychological Band-Aid. It is not counseling or psychotherapy. It can be learned by virtually any adult, even those without training in psychology. It is intended, however, for use by adults over age 21.

5) The E-PFA model, in its simplest form, consists of five dynamic and easy-to-remember processes, summarized in Table 1.1. In the rest of the book, we will expand on this summary and apply the processes to several types of psychological distress.

6) It is important to note that despite the best of intentions when trying to assist others, it is possible to inadvertently make things worse. Therefore, although this manual can be highly effective, we encourage pursuing more formal, structured training in PFA, just as you would to learn more about physical first aid. Part of this awareness and training includes recognizing when someone in distress requires more than PFA.

References

American Psychiatric Association. (1954). *Psychological first aid in community disasters.* American Psychiatric Association.

American Psychiatric Association. (2024). *New APA poll: One in three Americans feels lonely every week.* https://www.psychiatry.org/News -room/News-Releases/New-APA-Poll- One-in-Three-Americans -Feels-Lonely-Every-Week

American Red Cross. (2024). *Psychological first aid: Supporting yourself and others during COVID-19 online course.* https://www.redcross.org /take-a-class/coronovirus-information/psychological-first-aid -online-course

Ballard, J. (2019, July). *Millennials are the loneliest generation*. YouGov. https://today.yougov.com/society/articles/24577-loneliness -friendship-new-friends-poll-survey

Centers for Disease Control and Prevention. (2024, July). *Suicide data and statistics*. https://www.cdc.gov/suicide/facts/data.html

Deloitte Global. (2022). *The Deloitte Global 2022 Gen Z and Millennial Survey*. https://www.deloitte.com/global/en/issues/work/genz millennialssurvey-2022.htlm

Despeaux, K. E., Lating, J. M., Everly, G. S., Jr., Sherman, M. F., & Kirkhart, M. W. (2019). A randomized controlled trial assessing the efficacy of group psychological first aid. *Journal of Nervous and Mental Disease, 207*(8), 626–632. https://doi.org/10.1097/NMD.000000000001029

Durlak, J. (1979). Comparative effectiveness of paraprofessional and professional helpers. *Psychological Bulletin, 86*(1), 80–92. https://doi .org/10.1037/0033-2909.86.1.80

Editors. (2021, February). A psychological first aid kit. *Scientific American, 324*(2), 10. https://doi:10.1038/scientificamerican0221-10

Eisdorpher, C., & Golann, S. (1969). Principles of the training of "new professionals" in mental health. *Community Mental Health Journal, 5*, 349–357. https://doi.org/10.1007/BF01438980

Everly, G. S., Jr., Barnett, D. B., & Links, J. M. (2012). The Johns Hopkins model of psychological first aid (RAPID-PFA): Curriculum development and content validation. *International Journal of Emergency Mental Health, 14*(2), 95–103.

Everly, G. S., Jr., & Kennedy, C. (2019). Content validation of the Johns Hopkins model of psychological first aid (RAPID-PFA): Expanded curriculum. *Crisis, Stress, and Human Resilience, 1*(1) 6–14.

Everly, G. S., Jr., & Lating, J. M. (2022). *The Johns Hopkins guide to psychological first aid* (2nd ed.). Johns Hopkins University Press.

Everly, G. S., Jr., Lating, J. M., Sherman, M. F., & Goncher, I. (2016). The potential efficacy of psychological first aid on self-reported anxiety and mood: A pilot study. *Journal of Nervous and Mental Disease, 204*(3), 233–235. https://doi.org/10.1097/NMD.0000000000000429

Everly, G. S., Jr., McCabe, O. L., Semon, N., Thompson, C. B., & Links, J. (2014). The development of a model of psychological first aid (PFA) for non-mental health trained public health personnel: The Johns Hopkins' RAPID-PFA. *Journal of Public Health Management Practice, 2014, 20*(5), S24–S29. https://doi.org/10.1097/PHH.0000000000000065

Health Central (2024). Kevin Hines survived a jump off the Golden Gate Bridge—now he's helping others avoid suicide. https://www.healthcentral.com/condition/depression/kevin-hines-survived-golden-gate-bridge-suicide

Holt-Lunstad, J., Smith, T. B., Baker, M., Harris, T., & Stephenson, D. (2015). Loneliness and social isolation as risk factors for mortality: A meta-analytic review. *Perspectives on Psychological Science, 10*(2), 227–237. https://doi.org/10.1177/1745691614568352

Institute of Medicine. (2003). *Preparing for the psychological consequences of terrorism: A public health strategy.* National Academy of Sciences.

Jacobs, G. A. (2016). *Community-based psychological first aid.* Butterworth-Heineman.

McCabe, O. L., Everly, G. S., Jr., Brown, L. M., Wendelboe, A. M., Hamid, N. H. A., Tallchief, V. L., & Links, J. M. (2014). Psychological first aid: A consensus-derived, empirically supported, competency-based training model. *American Journal of Public Health, 104*(4), 621–628. https://doi.org/10.2105/AJPH.2013.301219

McCabe, O. L., Semon, N., Thompson, C. B., Lating, J. M., Everly, G. S., Jr., Perry, C. J., Moore, S. S., Mosley, A. M., & Links, J. (2014). Building a national model of public mental health preparedness and community resilience: Validation of a dual-intervention, systems-based approach. *Disaster Medicine and Public Health Preparedness, 8*(6), 511–526. https://doi.org/10.1017/dmp.2014.119

McGregor, D. (1960). *The human side of enterprise.* McGraw-Hill.

Ozer, E. J., Best, S. R., Lipsey, T. L., & Weiss, D. S. (2003). Predictors of posttraumatic stress disorder and symptoms in adults: A meta-analysis. *Psychological Bulletin, 129*(1), 52–73. https://doi.org/10.1037/0033-2909.1291.52

Pronovost, P., Berenholtz, S., Dorman, T., Lipsett, P. A., Simmonds, T., & Haraden C. (2003). Improving communication in the ICU using daily goals. *Journal of Critical Care, 18*(2), 71–75. https://doi.org. 10.1053/jcrc.2003.50008

Substance Abuse and Mental Health Administration (SAMHSA). (2015). *Core competencies for peer workers in behavioral health services.*

Winters, B. D., Gurses, A. P., Lehmann, H., Sexton, J. B., Rampersad, C. J., & Pronovost, P. J. (2009). Clinical review: Checklists—translating evidence into practice. *Critical Care, 13,* 210. https://doi.org/10.1186/cc7792

TWO | Everyday Psychological First Aid (E-PFA) Step-by-Step

ACCORDING TO THE AMERICAN RED CROSS (2024), psychological first aid (PFA) is "the practice of recognizing and responding to people experiencing crisis-related stress." It can help others (and oneself) cope with stressful events. This definition, while certainly accurate, leaves the reader wondering *how* it might be done.

If we go back in time in search of an answer, we discover a paper by F. C. Thorne published in the *Journal of Clinical Psychology* (Thorne, 1952). Dr. Thorne, a physician who also held a PhD in psychophysics, recognized two important realities: (1) There are times in almost everyone's life when stress becomes very challenging, if not unmanageable, and (2) as difficult as those moments may be, they do not require psychotherapy or psychiatric intervention. Thorne proposed a list of interventions, or active mechanisms, that he believed could be helpful in such circumstances: (1) offering reassurance, if possible, that things may not be as bad as they seem ("Everything's going to be okay"); (2) allowing people to talk about the circumstances and express their feelings (verbal catharsis or ventilation—talking it out); (3) providing suggestions for coping with the stress, depression, or tension.

According to the Institute of Medicine (2003), "Psychological first aid is a group of skills identified to limit distress and negative health behaviors. . . . PFA generally includes education about normal psychological responses to stressful and traumatic events; skills in active listening; understanding the importance of maintaining physical health and normal sleep, nutrition, and rest; and understanding when to seek help from professional caregivers" (p. 7).

After the terrorist attacks of September 11, 2001, and more recently the COVID-19 pandemic, interest in PFA increased dramatically as a way to help people cope with adversities. With a specific focus on public health emergencies and disasters, including terrorism, a PFA model known as RAPID was developed based on collaborations with the Johns Hopkins Center for Public Health Preparedness. Reports detailing the model's development were published beginning in the mid-1990s, with interest, as noted, increasing in the early 2000s (Everly et al., 2012; Everly & Flynn, 2006; Everly et al., 2006; Everly et al., 2014; McCabe, Everly, et al., 2014; McCabe, Semon, et al., 2014).

As described in Chapter One, the E-PFA model presented in this manual is derived from the original RAPID-PFA model and other sources, but has been adapted for broader use in households, workplaces, and community settings. It follows a checklist format outlining five phases (see Table 1.1). The model focuses on psychological distress and injuries (e.g., stress, grief, reactive depression, and other conditions), some of which most people are likely to encounter at least once in their lives. Other conditions, though less common, are still important to understand and prepare for.

Each chapter in Part Two of the manual addresses one of these conditions. These chapters are not meant to be read sequentially; rather, they are designed as stand-alone guides for understanding and addressing some of the most common forms of psychological distress or injury. This manual is intended to serve as a shelf reference for assisting with a range of psychological injuries, behavioral crises, and emergencies.

This chapter expands on the five-phase model introduced in Chapter One by filling in each phase with potential questions, suggestions, and prompts—its active ingredients or mechanisms of action—consistent with those recommended by Dr. Thorne. Before offering these components of E-PFA, however, it seems relevant to draw a parallel with the tools of physical first aid.

Tools for Physical First Aid

The generally recognized goals of physical first aid are to preserve life, prevent an injury from getting worse, reduce pain, and promote recovery. Medical science tells us that physical first aid employs a set of tools and interventions designed to assist individuals in acute physical distress. A standard first aid kit contains a variety of supplies, acknowledging that not all will be used at once:

1) Dressings such as Band-Aids and gauze wrap
2) Antiseptics
3) Antihistamines
4) Anti-inflammatories
5) Aspirin
6) Tweezers
7) Scissors
8) Step-by-step instructions for intervention processes, such as CPR, managing an arterial bleed, and providing assistance to someone who is choking (e.g., the Heimlich maneuver)

The skillful use of these tools is likely to reduce pain and promote healing, or at least delay the worsening of symptoms.

Tools for Everyday Psychological First Aid

The generally recognized goals of E-PFA are to preserve life (in cases where life is indeed in jeopardy), prevent a psychological injury from getting worse, reduce pain, and promote resilience, which may include seeking advanced support or care in the aftermath of problems, crises, or other adverse circumstances. As noted in the introduction to Part One, helping involves gathering information about what happened and the person's reactions to it, getting clarification, and then providing assistance. When considering how to offer support after gathering information and clarifying the situation, psychological research points to three core techniques commonly used in crisis intervention and stress management (Everly & Lating, 2019; Girdano & Everly, 1978; Lazarus, 1966; Lazarus & Folkman, 1984):

1) Problem-focused support: basic skills in mitigating or solving problems
2) Emotion-focused support: emotional ventilation, release, or expression (sometimes referred to as catharsis); and changing one's attitude or appraisal of the situation based on information and self-reflection
3) Stress response–focused support: stress management techniques and enlisting the support of others

With a slight modification, these coping techniques will form the basis of step four of the E-PFA model — providing assistance — throughout this manual. In this way, they become the key active ingredients of one's everyday psychological first aid kit.

A Simple E-PFA Model for Just About Anyone, Anywhere

As noted, the effectiveness of PFA may reside in its simplicity. To recap, our simplified E-PFA model consists of an easy-to-follow five-step formula: (1) Introduce the process and yourself (if necessary), (2) gather information, (3) clarify, (4) provide assistance, and (5) make a plan.

This section integrates the three core techniques from the previous section and shows how they can be applied using the following checklist of questions and suggestions. While not meant to be followed step-by-step, the checklist can be adapted to fit each situation and, in most instances, offers a helpful model for how the steps might flow.

1) "What happened?"
2) "What hurts?" (Or "How are you feeling about/reacting to what happened?")
3) "How bad is it?"
4) "What's the worst part of what happened?"
5) "What do you need most right now?" Other options, which may be used later, include: "What has helped you cope with stress in the past?" "What would you tell me if our roles were reversed?" The goal of asking these questions before rushing to solve problems is to foster resilience and to help the person in distress re-empower themselves.
6) "How can I help?"
7) Discuss options for reducing distress by focusing on the problem.
8) Discuss options for reducing distress by focusing on the emotional reactions.
9) Discuss options for reducing distress by focusing on the physical stress reactions.

10) What are the "next steps"? Make a plan to feel better. Discuss other resources.

The basic E-PFA formula, expanded with the above suggestions, is summarized in Table 2.1.

Table 2.1
E-PFA Step-by-Step

Introduce yourself, offer to help, and set expectations. Help de-escalate if needed.
This step is highly variable depending on whether or not you know the person. If you do not, you might simply say, "My name is _____. You look _____ (stressed, sad, out of it, etc.). Do you mind if I sit down? I'd like to help, if I can."

Gather information.
1)   Ask, "What happened?"
2)   Ask, "What hurts?" (Or "How are you feeling about what happened?" Questions such as "What reactions have you experienced?" or "what impact has this had on you so far?" can also be used.)
3)   Ask, "How bad is it?"

Clarify the main points.
4)   Check for the accuracy of what you've heard. Then ask, "What's the worst part of what happened?"

Provide options for assistance (select one or more).
5)   "What do you think would help you feel better or less distressed, at least right now?" "What have you done in the past to cope?" "What would you tell me to do if our roles were reversed?"
6)   "How can I help?" If nothing is requested, offer guidance/suggestions based on the following.
7)   Focus on the problem (situation). Can it be resolved or mitigated?
8)   Focus on the emotions. How can they best be mitigated?
9)   Focus on managing the stress response.

Make a plan.
10) Ask, "What are some good next steps?" Make a plan to help the person feel better. Questions like, "What can you do starting tomorrow to reduce the stress you are experiencing or to make things a little better?" can be useful. It's always a good idea to follow up to see if the acute distress has improved or to see if the person has acted on their plan to reduce stress.
   ○ Ask, "What other resources might be available to help with your plan (friends, family, etc.)?" Follow up, if possible.
   ○ Consider whether professional resources are needed.

In the next chapter we will delve even deeper into the five main components of the E-PFA kit.

KEY POINTS

1) According to the American Red Cross (2024), psychological first aid (PFA) is "the practice of recognizing and responding to people experiencing crisis-related stress." It can be used to help others—as well as oneself—cope in the face of stressful events.

2) This manual offers a simplified model of PFA—adapted from the RAPID model and others—to provide guidance for assisting individuals, family members, coworkers, and others.

3) Our E-PFA checklist consists of ten questions and suggestions (listed above) designed to foster emotional catharsis, facilitate introspection, and promote resilience.

References

American Red Cross. (2024). *Psychological first aid: Supporting yourself and others during COVID-19 online course.* https://www.redcross.org/take-a-class/coronavirus-information/psychological-first-aid-online-course.

Everly, G. S., Jr., Barnett, D. B., & Links, J. M. (2012). The Johns Hopkins model of psychological first aid (RAPID-PFA): Curriculum development and content validation. *International Journal of Emergency Mental Health, 14*(2), 95–103.

Everly, G. S., Jr., & Flynn, B. (2006). Principles and practical procedures for acute psychological first aid training for personnel without mental health experience. *International Journal of Emergency Mental Health, 8*, 93–100.

Everly, G. S., Jr., & Lating, J. M. (2019). *Clinical guide to the treatment of the human stress response* (4th ed.). Springer Nature.

Everly, G. S, Jr., McCabe, O. L., Semon, N., Thompson, C. B., & Links, J. (2014). The development of a model of psychological first aid (PFA) for non-mental health trained public health personnel: The Johns Hopkins' RAPID-PFA. *Journal of Public Health Management Practice, 20*(5), S24–S29. https://doi.org/10.1097/PHH.0000000000000065

Everly, G. S., Jr., Phillips, S., Kane, D., & Feldman, D. (2006). Introduction to and overview of group psychological first aid. *Brief Treatment and Crisis Intervention, 6*(2), 130–136. https://doi.org/10.1093/brief-treatment/mhj009

Girdano, D., & Everly, G. S., Jr. (1978). *Controlling stress and tension.* Prentice-Hall.

Institute of Medicine (2003). *Preparing for the psychological consequences of terrorism: A public health strategy.* National Academy of Sciences.

Lazarus, R. S. (1966). *Psychological stress and the coping process.* McGraw-Hill.

Lazarus, R. S., & Folkman, S. (1984). *Stress appraisal, and coping.* Springer.

McCabe, O. L., Everly, G. S., Jr., Brown, L. M., Wendelboe, A. M., Hamid, N. H. A., Tallchief, V. L., & Links, J. M. (2014). Psychological first aid: A consensus-derived, empirically supported, competency-based training model. *American Journal of Public Health, 104*(4), 621–628. https://doi.org/10.2105/AJPH.2013.301219

McCabe, O. L., Semon, N., Thompson, C. B., Lating, J. M., Everly, G. S., Jr., Perry, C. J., Moore, S. S., Mosley, A. M., & Links, J. (2014). Building a national model of public mental health preparedness and community resilience: Validation of a dual-intervention, systems-based approach. *Disaster Medicine and Public Health Preparedness, 8*(6), 511–526. https://doi.org/10.1017/dmp.2014.119

Thorne, F. C. (1952). Psychological first aid. *Journal of Clinical Psychology, 8*(2) 210–211. https://doi.org/10.1002/1097-4679(195204)8:2<210::aid-jclp2270080227>3.0.co;2-7

THREE | Everyday Psychological First Aid (E-PFA), Up Close and Personal

IN CHAPTER ONE, WE INTRODUCED the five-phase model of everyday psychological first aid (E-PFA). In Chapter Two, we added 10 questions and prompts that expand the model and bring it to life. These questions and suggestions are the *active ingredients*, or *mechanisms of action*, that help explain the model's impact in fostering calm and promoting resilience. In this chapter, we will take an even deeper dive into the mechanisms and provide background and additional resources.

Here is a recap of the five-phase formula:

1) Introduce yourself, offer to help, and set expectations. Help de-escalate if needed.
2) Gather information
3) Clarify and distill the main points you've heard.
4) Provide assistance.
5) Make a plan, and follow up if possible.

And here is a recap of the 10-step checklist that expands on the formula:

1) "What happened?"
2) "What hurts?" ("How are you feeling about what happened?")
3) "How bad is it?"
4) "What's the worst part of what happened?"
5) "What do you need most right now?"
6) "How can I help?"
7) Discuss options for reducing distress that focus on the problem.
8) Discuss options for reducing distress that focus on the person's emotional reactions.
9) Discuss options for reducing distress that focus on their physical reactions.
10) "What are some possible next steps?" Help them make a plan to feel better. Consider additional resources.

Table 2.1 from Chapter Two is replicated here as Table 3.1 for ease of reference.

According to Harvard psychiatry professor Theodore Millon (1999), the art of helping people in psychological distress consists of picking the best intervention at the right time for each unique person in each unique situation. E-PFA fits these criteria and can be used in a variety of circumstances. To reiterate, each E-PFA intervention is unique. You will choose the best form(s) of assistance for an individual in each specific situation and at the particular moment you encounter them.

The following descriptions of ways to assist are offered as lists of potential actions, not as a mandatory protocol. As useful as our manual may be, it is not intended to cover all possible situations. Rather, view it as a menu of options to be tailored to maximize effectiveness and avoid inadvertent harm.

Table 3.1
E-PFA Step-by-Step

Introduce yourself, offer to help, and set expectations. Help de-escalate if needed.
This step is highly variable depending on whether or not you know the person. If you do not, you might simply say, "My name is _____. You look _____ (stressed, sad, out of it, etc.). Do you mind if I sit down? I'd like to help, if I can."

Gather information.
1) Ask, "What happened?"
2) Ask, "What hurts?" (Or "How are you feeling about what happened?" Questions such as "What reactions have you experienced?" or "what impact has this had on you so far?" can also be used.)
3) Ask, "How bad is it?"

Clarify the main points.
4) Check for the accuracy of what you've heard. Then ask, "What's the worst part of what happened?"

Provide options for assistance (select one or more).
5) "What do you think would help you feel better or less distressed, at least right now?" "What have you done in the past to cope?" "What would you tell me to do if our roles were reversed?"
6) "How can I help?" If nothing is requested, offer guidance/suggestions based on the following.
7) Focus on the problem (situation). Can it be resolved or mitigated?
8) Focus on the emotions. How can they best be mitigated?
9) Focus on managing the stress response.

Make a plan.
10) Ask, "What are some good next steps?" Make a plan to help the person feel better. Questions like, "What can you do starting tomorrow to reduce the stress you are experiencing or to make things a little better?" can be useful. It's always a good idea to follow up to see if the acute distress has improved or to see if the person has acted on their plan to reduce stress.
    * Ask, "What other resources might be available to help with your plan (friends, family, etc.)?" Follow up, if possible.
    * Consider whether professional resources are needed.

Introduce Yourself, Offer to Help, Set Expectations, De-Escalate

In some cases, you may use E-PFA with people you do not know. In those instances, it's important to introduce yourself. (If you already know the person, clearly no introduction is necessary.)

Sometimes physical distress fuels psychological distress. In such cases, first address physical and safety needs as necessary. Offering physical first aid, providing water, walking away from a scene of crisis or conflict, or finding a quiet, safe place to talk can all be useful.

Offering to help someone in acute distress can be challenging. We are often unsure how to start the conversation. Fortunately, there is seldom a blatantly wrong approach—other than failing to offer help. Phrases like, "You look upset. How can I help? Do you mind if I sit down?" can start the conversation. Don't be surprised, though, if the person responds, "There's nothing you can do." In that case, you might say, *"Sometimes it helps to just talk about a problem. And if I can help, I will. If I can't, maybe I can find someone who can. How about we just chat?"* Informally setting expectations for how you might help can reduce some of the ambiguity in getting started.

Occasionally you will encounter someone who says, "Just leave me alone." In that situation, you might reply, *"Sometimes it helps to talk about a problem, but maybe this isn't the right time. I'm happy to just sit here with you if you want. You don't have to say anything."* If the person declines, you can simply say, "Okay, I'll check back with you later to see how you are doing."

Believe it or not, I (GSE) have used this approach while working with police, firefighters, and other rescuers in the rubble fields of the World Trade Center after the terrorist attacks of

September 11, 2001. I've also used it when helping my daughter after a challenging academic semester, and with a colleague facing a unique career challenge.

Be sure to adjust your approach and word choice to fit the person and the situation. A conversational tone is most effective, while a know-it-all or dismissive tone is, unsurprisingly, off-putting.

In some instances, the person you are trying to assist will be agitated or experiencing significantly heightened arousal. In those cases, the immediate focus shifts to psychological de-escalation, decompression, or "grounding."

In the context of E-PFA, de-escalation is the process of reducing acute psychological and physical arousal and ideally establishing a state of calm. It is critical to remember that the goal of de-escalation is not to solve the problem, but to lower the psychological and physical arousal that can block problem-solving or other crisis intervention. This is a form of psychological grounding.

Many psychological states or themes can increase arousal and agitation; the most frequently encountered are listed below. Listen for them. Identifying them can go a long way toward fostering empathy. Empathy—which can be thought of as similarity to or shared experience with another person—builds mutual understanding and, in turn, mutual trust.

Here are some common types of distress:

1) Frustration—caused by an action or goal that has been stifled or denied

2) Confusion—caused by receiving mixed messages or simply not understanding the message

3) Anger—hostility caused by some form of perceived insult or injury

4) Fear—apprehension about something anticipated to be harmful

5) Agitated reactive depression — due to a psychologically painful loss

6) Abandonment — being left out

7) Betrayal — over disloyalty by a trusted person

8) Ridicule — over having been bullied or humiliated

9) Guilt — over something done or not done

10) Grief — over loss

As long as someone remains in a highly aroused or defensive state, communication will be difficult, and problem-solving may be even more challenging, if not impossible.

What can you do to assist in de-escalation? De-escalation can be achieved through one or more of the following interventions. Remember, this is a list of options to be tailored uniquely and appropriately for each person and situation:

1) First, be sure the person is physically safe and not experiencing a medical crisis. When in doubt, assume that immediate physical assistance is needed, and respond accordingly.

2) Take a couple of deep breaths yourself, and project a calm demeanor. Diaphragmatic breathing (stomach breathing) is especially effective for lowering arousal (Lating et al., 2024). People tend to mimic the actions they see. Calm begets calm, anxiety begets anxiety. You can also ask the person in distress to take a few deep breaths.

3) Slow down the pace of your speech.

4) Always be respectful.

5) Avoid anything likely to be perceived as confrontational or aggressive (physically or psychologically), such as tone of voice or body posture (e.g., standing too close).

6) Acknowledge the person's distress. This allows them to express their emotions, whether it's anger, frustration, sadness, or fear. Saying something like, "You look really upset" can give them

implied permission to express their feelings. Don't be surprised if you get push-back, such as, "Well, how would you feel if this happened to you?" In that case, simply say something like, "Sorry, I'm just concerned."

7) Find a commonality or mutual interest, if such a sidebar conversation is appropriate or possible (e.g., residential area, hobbies, activities).

8) Use distraction if suitable. Physical distraction could entail asking the person to assist with a task (e.g., putting something away or moving an item). Psychological distraction might involve a simple counting exercise such as asking the person to count backward from 100 by twos, or backward from 30 by threes. You get the idea.

9) Use a grounding techniques such as the 3-3 method. Ask the person to choose three things to look at, one at a time, for about 30 seconds each. Have them focus on a spot on the wall, a tree, or a cloud—anything nondistressing. Then ask them to identify three things they can focus on touching or that may be touching them (e.g., their feet on the floor, the sensation of sitting or standing). Have then focus on each sensation for about 30 seconds. Repeat as needed. Grounding techniques are flexible, offering room to adjust both the number of objects and how long to focus on them.

10) Make use of clarifying questions. This shows interest and improves accuracy. "You said you were depressed. What does that feel like for you?"

11) Paraphrase important points of the conversation, and summarize them once the person has finished speaking. This can slow down the conversation while providing greater understanding. Ask them what they mean by a certain word or phrase.

12) Where appropriate, label emotions: "That sounds frustrating." "You look really upset."

13) Normalize the person's reactions, as appropriate. "It's understandable why you would be upset by this."

14) Provide reassurance, but do not make promises you cannot keep.

15) Correct any factual misconceptions fueling the distress. A simple correction, if accepted, can rapidly de-escalate arousal.

16) Remind the person they have options, even if the options are not ideal. Focusing on available choices, rather than threats of adverse consequences, can help ease distress by fostering a sense of control.

17) Suggest delaying any major decisions until a calmer state prevails.

18) If de-escalation fails and agitation persists, seek assistance as needed. This might include calling 9-1-1 if anyone's safety appears to be in jeopardy or if the situation grows into a medical emergency.

Gather Information

Gathering relevant information is usually a prerequisite to providing assistance. Be aware of the tendency to rush into fixing a problem that may not be readily or immediately solvable. It is a mistake to formulate a solution prior to fully understanding the situation. That's why gathering information is crucial.

As shown in Table 3.1, three simple questions (or similar ones) can assist in gathering relevant information about a psychological crisis:

1) "What happened?"
2) "What hurts?" (Or "How are you feeling about what happened?")
3) "How bad is it?"

Let's look at each question in turn.

When you encounter someone in acute distress, ask *what happened* to cause it. Without asking them to relive the experience, briefly determine the precipitating event or situation. Understanding the context will help you formulate an intervention plan. Vivid details are not essential, especially if recounting them would add to the person's distress.

The question "What hurts?" (psychologically speaking) continues the information-gathering process and helps identify the psychological or behavioral reactions that constitute the person's distress. The question "What hurts?" may be perceived by some as infantilizing, so asking "How are you feeling about this?" might be another choice. Observe how the stress is showing up. What thoughts, emotions, or actions indicate distress? Remember, not everyone experiences stress the same way.

Last, when you ask, *"How bad (severe) is it?"* think of severity as the combination of three factors: intensity, urgency, and duration. A simple formula may be useful:

Severity = Intensity + Urgency + Duration

Let's define each component.

Intensity. How disruptive is the distress? To what degree does it interfere with the person's ability to function daily? Consider asking, "How painful is your distress?"

Urgency. What is the degree to which the distress will worsen with time if not attended to? Urgency plus intensity usually indicates the priority for attention.

Duration. How long has the person experienced the distress?

Having defined the elements of severity, we can think of them as occupying a continuum ranging from mild to moderate to extreme.

Mild. Minimal interference with daily living. Low urgency. Duration could be short or long. Generally, the longer a person experiences psychological distress, even mild, the more problematic it becomes.

Moderate. Some interference with desired activities, but little or no disruption to essential activities of daily life. Urgency stems from a desire to feel better but lacks desperation. Duration may be short or long.

Extreme. Significant interference with essential activities. Significant risk of worsening distress and dysfunction if not addressed. Duration may be short or long.

As you will see in Part Two of the manual, many of the severity questions will be incorporated into the E-PFA recommendations and dialogues. The detailed explanation provided here is meant to offer a helpful framework for understanding severity.

Clarify and Distill

After the person in distress has described what happened, how they are reacting, and the severity of their distress, pause for a moment and paraphrase the key points you've heard. A paraphrase involves restating to the person what you've heard—about their thoughts, feelings, and/or actions—in your own words. The goal is to add clarity, check for accuracy, and offer empathy. We will discuss the paraphrase in more detail in Chapter Four.

Most people who are new to psychological first aid ask, "Where do I begin?" Once you've paraphrased what you've heard, you can ask a simple question to identify a starting place for your assistance: *"What's the worst part of all this?"* This helps you pinpoint where to focus your efforts, at least initially.

To summarize:

1) Use paraphrasing to seek greater detail and to confirm accuracy of what you're hearing.
2) Ask, "What's the worst part of all this?" to help distill facts and reveal a starting point for psychological assistance.

Provide Assistance

Begin with exploratory questions like, *"What do you need most right now?"* Other questions that can be used later in the process might include, *"What have you done to manage stress in the past?"* or *"What would you tell me if our situations were reversed?"* The question *"How can I help?"* can follow these or stand on its own.

These broad, open-ended questions are designed to help the person in distress tap into their own resilience and determine if there is something you can do to assist in a straightforward manner. The focus should be on the immediate moment, not the long term. Remember, this is first aid, not psychotherapy.

If the person doesn't know how you can help, validate their reactions and consider recommending options to foster coping and resilience, such as the more directed approaches listed below.

Based on the research of Lazarus and Folkman (1984) and others (Girdano & Everly, 1978), and as noted in Chapter Two and Table 3.1, providing direct assistance can entail one or more of three processes:

1) Problem-focused assistance
2) Emotion-focused assistance
3) Stress reaction–focused assistance

Problem-Focused Assistance

Possible questions:

"How can the problem be solved?"
"What has to happen to make this problem go away?"
"What can be done to make the problem less severe?"

Logic dictates that if psychological distress is associated with an external problem or incident, the easiest solution is to solve the problem. Thus, a problem-focused intervention is worth considering. To help the person help themselves, you can ask, *"How can the problem be solved?"* or *"What has to happen to make this problem go away?"* These questions aim to identify potential remedies and foster a sense of empowerment.

Understand, however, that in many instances the problem cannot be solved, but its severity can be mitigated. In that case, you can ask, *"What can be done to make the problem less severe?"* Again, the focus of the intervention is on the external problem or situation.

The Chinese philosopher Confucious once asserted that insight is gained and problems are solved or mitigated through three methods: imitation, experience, and self-reflection/introspection. Twenty-five hundred years later, psychological science has confirmed these approaches. They can be organized into a three-step process:

1) *Imitation.* Social learning models (Bandura, 1997) confirm that learning and problem-solving often begin through observation and imitation. A person in distress who wants to lose bad habits and acquire healthier ones might benefit from observing and speaking with those who have done something similar. This applies to issues ranging from relationship discord to career challenges to health problems (both physical and mental). Hotlines and support groups exist for almost every situation, offering role

models who have "been there and done that," and who can assist with problem-solving, resilience, and growth. If you want your children to learn to solve problems and manage stress, help them form friendships with people who do those things well. If you want your supervisees to handle pressure effectively, place them among people who have learned to do so.

2) *Experience.* Experiencing new behaviors firsthand by imitating role models becomes a powerful teacher. New behaviors are either extinguished or sustained under what are known in behavioral psychology as the laws of operant conditioning. Here, the work of the influential psychologist E. L. Thorndike (1927, 1933) becomes relevant. His Law of Effect states that behaviors followed by a positive outcome—that is, reinforced in some way—are more likely to be repeated, while behaviors followed by a negative outcome are less likely to be repeated. As obscure as it may sound, the Law of Effect is essential knowledge for everyday life, especially for parents, teachers, and managers. It explains why people do many of the things they do, including behaviors that may seem to make no sense. In reality, human behavior almost always makes sense to the person performing the action, even if others fail to understand it. If an action is repeated, it means that somehow, in some way, it is rewarding—by either helping the person get something they want or helping them avoid something they don't want.

3) *Self-reflection/introspection.* According to Confucious, Aristotle, and others, this is the most noble road to wisdom and problem-solving. Informed self-reflection not only can reveal new options; it can also help remove barriers to growth. The most powerful reinforcement comes from within. Answers we arrive at ourselves—or can genuinely endorse after contemplation—are far more likely to be accepted and followed. Analyst Carl Jung once observed that those who look outside themselves dream, while those who look inside themselves awaken.

Confucious and Aristotle gave us these overarching processes for insight and problem-solving, but it was the Greek philosopher Socrates, considered the greatest teacher of his era, who provided a fundamental heuristic—a strategy to help people solve problems and make quick, efficient decisions—that led to specific intervention tactics. This heuristic is the foundation of the famous Socratic dialogues. Although using the dialogues is not always practical in daily situations, we offer the following checklist for solving and mitigating problems, adapted from the Socratic method:

1) State the problem.
2) Identify its cause.
3) Distill the essence of the problem. Why is the situation a problem, or what lies at the core of the problem?
4) Identify the current and future effects of the problem.
5) Consider ways to solve the problem.
6) Evaluate the best-case and worst-case scenarios for solving it.
7) Consider ways to lessen (mitigate) its severity.
8) Evaluate the best-case and worst-case scenarios for lessening its severity.
9) Implement the solution or mitigation plan.
10) Evaluate.

Emotion-Focused Assistance

Possible questions:

"What would help you feel better right now?"
"What are you saying to yourself about this situation that's making it so stressful?"
"What could you say to yourself that would lessen some of that stress?"
"What things have helped you feel better in the past?"

"What would you tell me if our roles (or situations) were reversed?"

Do not be surprised if you discover that the problem itself cannot be resolved or mitigated. Some problems (e.g., diagnosis of a chronic illness, or an unchangeable event) cannot be fixed and must instead be endured. In such cases, the focus shifts from the external problem to the internal distress being experienced. Most of this manual focuses not on problem-solving but on reducing distress and fostering resilience associated with problems that are not easily remedied.

In an effort to help the person help themselves, you can ask, *"What has helped you feel better in the past?"* Reminding them of techniques they have used successfully before can reduce feelings of helplessness. According to Socrates, mobilizing the potency of self-empowering questions is preferable to offering suggestions or options right away.

Whether in the form of questions or suggestions, psychologists have identified what may be the single most powerful tool for reducing acute distress. This collection of techniques—often called "rational thinking" or, more formally, "cognitive reappraisal," "cognitive restructuring," or "cognitive reinterpretation"—asserts a clear idea: Our thoughts control our emotions; therefore, by changing our thoughts we can greatly affect our emotions. Research and clinical applications—from Albert Bandura's work in self-efficacy (Bandura, 1997), to Albert Ellis's prescriptions for rational thinking (Ellis & Harper, 1979), to Aaron Beck's psychiatric applications of cognitive therapy (Beck, 1976), and David Burns's popularization of that work (Burns, 1980)—all emphasize the power of thought and attitude to affect human emotions, especially stress.

This notion is not new. In fact, it was a core tenet of the Stoic philosophers of ancient Greece, who asserted that people are disturbed not by things, but by the views they take of them. In a different context, John Milton wrote in *Paradise Lost*, "The mind is its own place and in itself / Can make a Heaven of Hell, a Hell of Heaven." Perhaps one of the most compelling endorsements of this idea came from the father of the stress concept himself. Hans Selye, a brilliant endocrinologist and experimental surgeon who coined the term "stress" in the biological sciences, wrote in his famous book *The Stress of Life* (1956), "It's not what happens to you that matters. It's how you take it." If these assertions are true, as we believe they are, imagine the power one has by simply changing one's mind. This power can be harnessed in E-PFA, as promoted in *Cognitive Behavioral Strategies in Crisis Intervention* (Dattilio & Freeman, 1994).

Albert Ellis, mentioned above, was an American psychologist who suggested that psychological support should be practical and focus on conscious thought. He developed the A-B-C-D model, which emphasizes the power of thoughts, attitudes, and interpretations. Ellis (and others) asserted that adverse external events and situations (A) do not directly cause undesirable consequences (C) like stress, depression, and anxiety (see figure below).

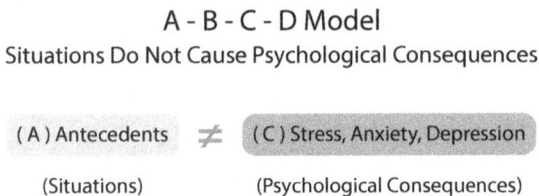

A - B - C - D Model
Situations Do Not Cause Psychological Consequences

(A) Antecedents   ≠   (C) Stress, Anxiety, Depression

(Situations)   (Psychological Consequences)

Rather, the culprit is the belief (B), or *what we say to ourselves* about events, that causes psychological distress (see figure below).

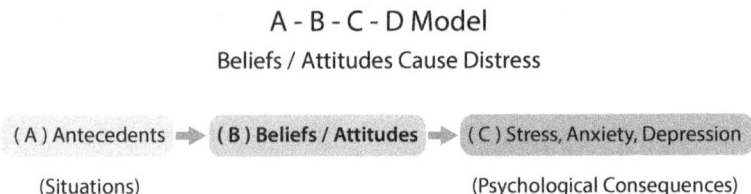

A - B - C - D Model
Beliefs / Attitudes Cause Distress

(A) Antecedents ➡ (B) Beliefs / Attitudes ➡ (C) Stress, Anxiety, Depression

(Situations)   (Psychological Consequences)

The implication for E-PFA is clear: Emotion-focused assistance entails helping people discover *what they are saying to themselves* about the situation, and then disputing (D) worst-case-scenario thinking or correcting beliefs that are clearly wrong, unsupported by evidence, or what some might call "irrational."

From an E-PFA perspective, listen carefully as people tell their stories, and watch for assumptions that are not necessarily backed by evidence. When a person in distress describes the "worst part" of a situation, you can simply ask, "Are you sure the outcome will be so severe?" or "What is the evidence?" Even if the negative consequences are realistic, promoting optimism and helping the person regain a sense of control can be very effective in reducing anxiety, stress, depression, and even traumatic stress (see figure below).

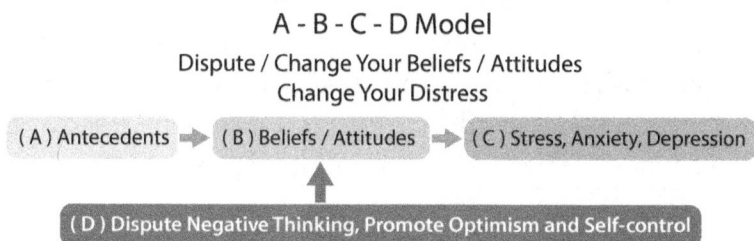

A - B - C - D Model
Dispute / Change Your Beliefs / Attitudes
Change Your Distress

(A) Antecedents ➡ (B) Beliefs / Attitudes ➡ (C) Stress, Anxiety, Depression

⬆

(D) Dispute Negative Thinking, Promote Optimism and Self-control

A subtle and more indirect way to encourage a person to question their own pessimism and think more optimistically is through a form of indirect self-reflection. Ask, *"What would you tell me if our roles (or situations) were reversed?"* Remember that a person in crisis — adolescents as well as adults — feel out of control, and what they often want most is to regain a sense of control. Merely giving them options may be less effective than asking what advice they would recommend if *you* were in distress. This approach fosters self-reflection in a less direct, more accessible way. It can also be used at the beginning of this phase, as outlined in Table 3.1.

Stress Response–Focused Assistance

Possible questions:

> "What stress management techniques have you successfully used
>   in the past?"
> "Do you mind if I offer some information or other options?"

Stress response–focused assistance involves offering concrete options for managing physical and psychological stress arousal. Before doing so, you might ask what stress management techniques have worked for the person in the past. (This question can also be used earlier in the phase.) If it does not generate a useful response, consider asking, *"Do you mind if I offer some information or other options?"* At that point, you can offer specific stress management strategies not already discussed.

Information and guidance are typically provided in three forms: explanatory guidance, anticipatory guidance, and prescriptive guidance. Let's take a look at each.

Explanations or information (explanatory guidance) can help normalize the person's experience and reassure them that their reactions are common given the circumstances they've faced. Sometimes explanatory guidance is offered as a way of simply explaining what the underlying cause of the felt distress might be.

Anticipations or warnings (anticipatory guidance) help shape expectations and can include warnings like, "You may have difficulty sleeping for a while," or "You may find yourself more irritable." These are usually based on experiences the helper has encountered or witnessed.

Suggestions (prescriptive guidance) include recommendations for coping and stress management. Many effective techniques exist for managing stress and fostering resilience. Everly and Lating (2019) have conducted thorough reviews and provided step-by-step guidelines for implementing these techniques:

1) Physical exercise
2) Nutrition
3) Rest and sleep hygiene
4) Writing in a journal
5) Recruiting the support of friends and family

The following list goes into greater detail (American Academy of Sleep Medicine, 2016; Everly & Lating, 2019; McCann & Everly, 2024). Bear in mind that it is generally wise to check with a qualified health care professional before altering one's diet or exercise.

1) Regular *moderate* physical exercise offers the following benefits. (Exercise that is extreme—in intensity or duration—can be dangerous as it may increase the risk of injury or cardiopulmonary distress.)
   a. Improves self-confidence and self-esteem
   b. Reduces depression
   c. Improves endurance and strength (if resistance is used)
   d. Improves learning
   e. Improves sleep
   f. Helps with weight control
   g. Promotes relaxation for several hours following exercise
2) Think of nutrition as fuel for daily living.
   a. Eating six smaller meals appears to be preferable to eating three larger meals totaling the same calories.
   b. Energy drinks typically contain stimulants for the central nervous system, which, while temporarily increasing strength and endurance, can also strain the heart and

increase blood pressure. Energy drinks can be physiologically and psychologically addicting.

   c. Sometimes depression can lead to a reduction in appetite. Maintaining a healthy diet is usually recommended despite loss of appetite.

   d. Some vitamins and herbal supplements can have health-promoting and even stress-reducing effects. Some herbal supplements can even aid sleep. But caution must be taken, as there are no herbal magic bullets to eliminate stress. And some supplements can interfere with the actions of prescription medications.

3) Rest and sleep are when the body and mind repair and restore themselves.

   a. Adolescents require 8 to 10 hours of sleep every 24 hours.

   b. Adults require 7 hours of sleep every 24 hours.

   c. A 20- to 30-minute nap improves cognitive capacity and can partially compensate for lost sleep.

   d. The practice of techniques that promote a relaxation response (such as mindfulness, meditation, and imagery) has been shown to reduce stress, improve healing, and help develop a lasting sense of calm.

   e. Consistent inadequate sleep has been associated with the development of dementia.

4) Consider writing in a journal.

   a. Dr. James Pennebaker (1999) has studied the power of self-disclosure, especially through writing, and has found it to be an effective tool for promoting health and managing stress.

   b. Keeping a daily record of thoughts, emotions, and actions is not only cathartic; it can educate, motivate, and heal.

   c. Journaling also seems to improve physical health.

5) Interpersonal support has been shown to be a powerful predictor of resilience. Encouraging the person to enlist the support of friends and family can be a recommendation for this phase, or it can be incorporated into making a plan (next phase).

Make a Plan

Make a plan for next steps. It's often said that if something doesn't get scheduled, it won't get done. Give the person practical "homework" to begin fostering resilience. Planning is also a form of empowerment, as it implies hope, optimism, and an investment of time and energy. Start with a question like, *"What can you do to begin to help yourself feel better?"* or *"What has helped you in the past?"* or *"So, where do we go from here?"* or *"What can you do beginning tomorrow to help yourself feel better?"*

Given the acute nature of the psychological Band-Aid that E-PPA represents, it is often wise to suggest that anyone enduring a crisis, regardless of its magnitude, reach out for continued support. Research shows that support from others is one of the most effective ways to foster resilience (Cohen & Hoberman, 1983; Dinenberg et al., 2014; Ozer et al., 2003; Wang et al., 2018). As the Roman philosopher and statesman Cicero noted, friends multiply happiness and divide sadness. Professional resources—such as primary health care practitioners, psychologists, psychiatrists, and faith-based support—may also be valuable. Encourage the person to reach out to friends, family, coworkers, and/or professionals. In doing so, resilience can be fostered and growth promoted.

Try to follow up if possible. If you've given them "homework," check in to see how it's going. Follow up in and of itself shows you care, regardless of whether they are known to you or are a stranger.

KEY POINTS

1) This chapter takes a deeper dive into each of the five phases of E-PFA and their active ingredients.

2) The easiest form of psychological crisis intervention is often problem-solving, as the stressor simply goes away—a relief all of us have experienced. If a problem cannot be solved, it can often be mitigated, making it more manageable and significantly reducing the distress it causes. This chapter provides checklist approaches for solving and mitigating problems.

3) Problem-solving and mitigation can be delayed or inhibited by psychological and physical arousal. People cannot focus on solutions—no matter how obvious they seem to others—until their stress levels decline. Therefore, it's important to apply simple de-escalation techniques first. This chapter provides a checklist of de-escalation interventions to choose from.

4) The three questions used to gather information are: (a) What happened? (b) What hurts? (c) How bad is it?

5) A clear-cut formula for assess the severity of a crisis is: Severity = Intensity + Urgency + Duration.

6) When clarifying and distilling information about a situation, asking about its worst aspect can be helpful.

7) Providing assistance generally falls into three categories: (a) problem-focused, (b) emotion-focused, and (c) stress response–focused.

8) It's important to make a plan for next steps and, if possible, to follow up. Part of that plan should entail encouraging the person to reach out to others—friends, family, coworkers, or professional resources—for support.

9) E-PFA is not counseling or psychotherapy. It is a psychological Band-Aid. You might make one or two contacts to help reduce acute distress and to "jump-start" efforts toward resilience. The

processes described in this manual offer a menu of options to help reduce distress; they are not cures.

References

American Academy of Sleep Medicine. (2016). *Teen sleep duration health advisory.* https://aasm.org/advocacy/position-statements/teen-sleep-duration-health-advisory/

Bandura, A. (1997). *Self-efficacy: The exercise of control.* W. H. Freeman.

Beck, A. (1976). *Cognitive therapy and the emotional disorders.* International Universities Press.

Burns, D. (1980). *Feeling good: The new mood therapy.* Morrow.

Cohen, S., & Hoberman, H. M. (1983). Positive events and social supports as buffers of life change stress. *Journal of Applied Social Psychology, 13*(2), 99–125. https://doi.org/10.1111/j.1559-1816.1983.tb02325.x

Dattilio, F. M., & Freeman, A. (1994). *Cognitive behavioral strategies in crisis intervention.* Guilford.

Dinenberg, R. E., McCaslin, S. E., Bates, M. N., & Cohen, B. E. (2014). Social support may protect against development of posttraumatic stress disorder: Findings from the Heart and Soul Study. *American Journal of Health Promotion, 28*(5), 294–297. https://doi.org/10.4278/ajhp.121023-QUAN-511

Ellis, A., & Harper, R. A. (1979). *A new guide to rational living.* Wilshire Book Co.

Everly, G. S., Jr., & Lating, J. M. (2019). *A clinical guide to the treatment of the human stress response* (4th ed.). Springer Science & Business Media.

Girdano, D., & Everly, G. S., Jr. (1978). *Controlling stress and tension.* Prentice-Hall.

Lating, J. M., Everly, G. S., Jr., Sherman, M. F., Kennedy-Dunn, C. M., & Quinn, L. C. (2024). Frontalis muscle electromyographic (EMG) biofeedback-assisted relaxation training: A novel approach for developing stress resistance. *Crisis, Stress, and Human Resilience: An International Journal, 5*(4), 131–144.

Lazarus, R. S., & Folkman, S. (1984). *Stress: Appraisal and coping.* Springer.

McCann, J., & Everly, G. S., Jr. (2024). *Lodestar: Tapping into the ten timeless pillars to success*. Simon and Schuster.

Millon, T. (1999). *Personality guided therapy*. Wiley.

Ozer, E. J., Best, S. R., Lipsey, T. L., & Weiss, D. S. (2003). Predictors of posttraumatic stress disorder and symptoms in adults: A meta-analysis. *Psychological Bulletin, 129*(1), 52–73. https://doi.org/10.1037/0033-2909.129.1.52

Pennebaker, J. (1999) The effects of traumatic disclosure on physical and mental health: The values of writing and talking about upsetting events. *International Journal of Emergency Mental Health, 1*(1), 9–18.

Selye, H. (1956). *The stress of life*. McGraw-Hill.

Thorndike, E. L. (1927). The law of effect. *American Journal of Psychology, 39*, 212–222. https://doi.org/10.2307/1415413

Thorndike, E. L. (1933). A proof of the law of effect. *Science, 77*, 173–175. https://doi.org/10.1126/science.77.1989.173.b

Wang, L., Tao, H., Bowers, B. J., Brown, R., & Zhang, Y. (2018). Influence of social support and self-efficacy on resilience of early career registered nurses. *Western Journal of Nursing Research, 40*(5), 648–664. https://doi.org/10.1177/0193945916685712

FOUR

The Power of Compassionate
Communication

If you just communicate, you can get by. But if you
communicate skillfully, you can work miracles.

—JOHN ROHN

"COMMUNICATION — OR A LACK THEREOF — can
make the difference between success and failure. Effective communication can inspire others to action,
make a process go smoothly, and plant the seeds for
new ways of thinking." This quote from the homepage
of the University of Southern California's Annenberg
School for Communication captures the essential role
communication plays. What more powerful tool could
someone practicing E-PFA ask for? Compassionate
communication is the medium through which E-PFA
exerts its stress-reducing influence, starting with establishing rapport. It forms the foundation for each of
the five phases of the E-PFA model and lies at the heart
of every applied chapter in Part Two of this manual.

The Nuts and Bolts of Communication

Studies have shown that communication has three core elements: the sender, the receiver, and the message. In E-PFA communications, you will be the sender. The person experiencing distress will be the receiver. The message will vary from situation to situation, but it must always convey compassion and support, embedded in the five steps of E-PFA. Let's examine each of the core elements of crisis communication.

The Sender

E-PFA starts before you say anything; it begins with presence. Presence can be thought of as "showing up." It's your physical and emotional availability and appearance. Sometimes that's what a person in distress needs most. And sometimes it's all they need. Whether in person, online, or over the phone, presence matters. Some have referred to this as a "ministry of presence." In this context, "ministry" does not imply a religious role, but rather a caring attentiveness toward another person.

Often, however, mere presence is not enough. The type of presence matters. Displaying calmness and some degree of self-confidence under pressure (not arrogance, and especially not dismissiveness) can be an important aspect of an effective ministry of presence, especially in situations where the person in distress or experiencing a psychological injury feels out of control or fearful. Do not underestimate this skill; demonstrating calmness and confidence during an adverse situation sends a powerful, soothing, and even reassuring message.

Consider the following scenario. Amber received a call from a friend, Emily, who was in significant distress over the loss of a loved one. Amber drove to Emily's house. On the way there she kept thinking about what to say. Amber, who grew up in a close-knit family with traditional family values, assumed that the loss of a loved one would affect Emily as it would her. So Amber assumed that Emily would be devastated. When Amber arrived, Emily was clearly distressed but not devastated, as Amber had assumed she would be. Amber was unsure what to say or do. She simply said, "I'm so sorry. What can I do?" Emily replied, "There's nothing, but thanks." For the next hour Amber and her friend sat together in silence. In the meantime, other friends gathered to support Emily.

Amber left feeling as though she had let Emily down. She knew she hadn't "solved" the problem. She hadn't made her friend feel any better. But how could she? Two days later Amber received a note from Emily: "Dearest Amber, Thanks for all you did, I will never ever forget it." What did Amber do? She showed up. She was present, and her caring, compassionate, nonintrusive presence genuinely mattered to Emily.

Values and Assumptions

Any preexisting values and assumptions you hold about either the person in distress or the situation can impact your effectiveness as a communicator. A preexisting value, psychologically speaking, refers to the importance, worth, or general emotional valence (positive or negative) you assign to a person, place, action, or thing. Some people, for example, struggle to help someone else who has done something risky or inappropriate, believing that the person "got what they deserve." But E-PFA does not involve passing judgment; it is about helping someone in distress.

Assumptions are preconceived conclusions made in the absence of direct evidence. It is common to rely on assumptions during listening to "fill in the gaps" in someone's story rather than taking the time to ask for clarification. Assumptions can speed up the process — but what if they are incorrect? How many times have you miscommunicated because you assumed something about a person or situation that turned out to be false? Sometimes the assumptions we make say more about us than about the other person. Values and assumptions can serve as filters, interfering with your objectivity and ability to remain fully present. Recognizing and managing them is an important and ongoing part of the E-PFA process.

The Receiver (Person in Distress)

A key aspect of communication is speaking in a way the other person can understand. It helps to consider what someone in distress might be experiencing. Often, there are three overarching reactions, sometimes referred to as the crisis triad (Everly & Mitchell, 2008):

1) Feelings of uncertainty and perhaps loss of control and pessimism about the future.
2) Impaired ability to think clearly or logically (sometimes called a "dumbing down" reaction or, more formally, cortical inhibition)
3) A tendency toward impulsive action

It is essential to keep these reactions in mind when communicating with someone in crisis, as they can interfere with your overall effectiveness.

To help you initially connect with someone, remember that human communication occurs both verbally and nonverbally, and involves both cognitive (or intellectual) and emotional dimensions. Under normal circumstances, most people lead with their heads (thinking/cognitive faculties) and follow with their hearts (emotional faculties). We all know people who are exceptions; they lead with their hearts or wear their emotions on their sleeve. But during or in the immediate wake of a crisis, most people, regardless of their usual style, communicate primarily through emotional expression, or the intentional suppression of emotions. In these moments, rational thought is often compromised, while confusion or distraction is often evident.

This point is important to keep in mind when administering E-PFA. Do your best to gauge whether the person in crisis is leading with their head or their heart. Intellectual or thinking-based messages will likely be ineffective for someone consumed by emotion, while emotionally charged messages may not resonate with a person using an analytic approach to coping (or trying to suppress their emotions). Those leading with their heads are typically seeking information, whereas those leading with their hearts are usually seeking emotional support. When providing E-PFA, aim to match your approach to the immediate needs of the person in crisis. And be aware that the person in crisis may be inclined to act impulsively.

The Message

Let's take a closer look at the two forms of communication: nonverbal and verbal.

Nonverbal Communication

Mark Twain once noted that actions speak louder than words. Research shows that this bit of wisdom has some validity. Nonverbal communication—in the form of body language (facial expressions, hand gestures, other bodily movements) and paralinguistics (tone or how the words are said, speech rate, etc.)—has been demonstrated in laboratory studies to account for a significant portion of the message being communicated (Mehrabian, 1971). Therefore, when applying E-PFA, it is crucial to be mindful of the message your nonverbal behavior sends. Additionally, it's important to monitor the nonverbal communication of the person in crisis.

Here are a few things to consider:

- The firmness and reassurance of your handshake (if you shake hands)
- Establishing and maintaining comfortable eye contact
- Sitting with an open and receptive posture (arms unfolded, legs uncrossed, body leaning slightly forward)
- Maintaining a safe and comfortable interpersonal distance
- Staying attentive (not appearing distracted, even if there are possible distractions)
- Facial expressions (e.g., nodding affirmatively, avoiding frowning or yawning)
- Minimizing foot and leg movement

Be aware that there are optimal levels for most nonverbal behaviors. For example, too much eye contact might be perceived as staring, and excessive head nodding or other movement can be distracting.

When considering others' nonverbal behaviors, pay attention to the following signals they may convey:

- Handshake — is it passive, cold, or sweaty, indicating a sympathetic nervous system response, or extremely tight, indicating a lack of awareness or desperate efforts to control the situation?
- Willingness and ability to maintain eye contact
- Evidence of the "thousand-yard stare," which is can be brought on by stressful events, causing the person to block out or minimize their surroundings and stare off into "nothing"
- Facial expressions (e.g., blank, tearful, frowning)
- Seated posture (e.g., slouched as if exasperated, arms folded, suggesting defensiveness)
- Body movements (e.g., shaking legs, suggesting anxiousness)

Be mindful of cultural differences and norms when assisting others. For example, some groups consider sustained eye contact offensive or disrespectful, or may avoid eye contact when talking about serious topics (Brammer & MacDonald, 1996; Ivey, 1994). Additionally, North American and British people generally prefer more physical distance during conversation than people from many other cultures.

Verbal Communication: The Use of Statements

When encountering a receiver (i.e., person in crisis), many of us, including the authors upon occasion, tend to respond by immediately telling them what they should do to solve a problem or cope better. While such responses certainly seem logical, research suggests that a more effective initial approach is to ask questions before providing answers. Why? Most receivers do not want to be "rescued," per se. Rather, they first want to be heard, they want to vent, and often they want to regain a sense of control. Rushing to solve someone's problem can deprive them of that empowering, confidence-building process. This may lead to frustration, as the receiver might feel the sender doesn't understand. Problem-solving and offering coping options may be better received after some time has passed, when the receiver realizes that assistance really is necessary. Solution-oriented statements and suggestions usually come in the last phase of the E-PFA model, providing assistance (see Chapter Three).

Verbal Communication: The Use of Questions

Questions are used throughout all phases of the E-PFA model, but especially in the gathering information phase. They can be used for initial inquiry, to seek clarification, and even to foster introspection or reflection in the providing assistance phase. They can "jump start" a process of regaining self-control.

There are generally two types of questions: closed-ended and open-ended. These are broad categories, and there is a rationale for when and why each is used in PFA. Closed-ended questions ask for specific information and limit the response options. The most restrictive closed-ended questions are those that elicit a "yes" or "no" reply. Common examples of closed-ended stems include: "Do you . . . ?" "Don't you . . . ?" "Is this . . . ?" "Isn't this . . . ?" "Was it . . . ?" The sender should be careful not to use too many closed-ended questions in a row, particularly if they might be perceived as probing or interrogative by the receiver. So, we see closed-ended questions can be used to confirm an assumption or a previous statement.

Conversely, open-ended questions are exploratory and encourage the person to provide more information. Stems for open-ended questions include: "Who," "What," "How," "When," "Where," "Why." However, it's generally best to limit the use of "why" questions early on, as they can make the other person feel judged and may increase defensiveness. E-PFA senders should also avoid using too many open-ended questions in succession, as this can unintentionally signal that they are not truly listening. Paraphrasing, discussed below, can be used to break up a series of open-ended questions and demonstrate active listening.

Understanding the benefits of both closed-ended and open-ended questions can be very helpful in crisis situations. Closed-ended questions can be useful for helping someone transition from intense emotional expression to a more cognitive state. Moreover, as described above, people in crisis may struggle to think clearly in a crisis. Asking deeply probing or highly personal questions too soon might exacerbate this difficulty. Such questions are usually inappropriate for any type of crisis intervention. It is often more effective to begin with closed-ended questions or observational statements, such as, "You look like you are having a hard time," and then move to open-ended, exploratory questions like, "So, what's going on?"

Reflective statements and paraphrasing help demonstrate that you, the sender, are truly present and listening. Let's look at how to use them effectively in E-PFA.

Reflective Listening Techniques: Restatements and Paraphrasing

The second phase and especially the third phase of the E-PFA model hinges on reflective listening, as this is where you check the accuracy of what you have heard. These are often referred to as "mirroring" techniques because they reflect back what the person is saying without adding interpretation or judgment. While several such techniques exist, we will focus on restatement and paraphrasing.

The primary goals of reflective listening—and the third phase of our model—are to: (1) clarify ambiguities, (2) distill thoughts and feelings into a core theme, and (3) help the other person feel understood. Remember that understanding creates trust. But remember you should always seek clarification when you do not understand something that has been said, regardless of what phase of the model you are in.

The most basic reflective techniques are nonverbal or paraverbal. To help someone in distress express their stress, frustration, anger, or sadness, use simple, socially reinforcing or minimally encouraging words like, "Uh-huh," "Hmm," "Yeah," "I see," or "Really?" Placing these brief responses at the end of a receiver's statement or during a pause can convey empathy and signal that you are yielding your turn to talk, encouraging the receiver to continue. Overusing this tool can, however, come across as distracting or even dismissive.

Another key reflective listening technique is restatement. Restatements repeat back the receiver's own words, usually in a more concise form, to concretely and clearly highlight the relevance of what they said. They serve as a check for accurate listening and give the receiver a moment to pause and reflect on what they are saying—a particularly salient process in a crisis, when overwhelming emotions and cortical inhibition might lead to confused thinking. Accurate restatements help the person hear how their concerns sound to others. For example: "You used the word 'sad' to describe how you've been feeling." As with other techniques, overuse of restatement can be distracting, making it seem as thought you are parroting rather than really listening.

One of the most commonly used, and perhaps most powerful, reflective technique is the summary paraphrase. The goal of a summary paraphrase is to capture and reflect back, in your own words, the important points of what was just said, but in a more concise form. A summary paraphrase might be used when the receiver pauses or finishes speaking. It allows the receiver continue with minimal interruption while signaling that they are being heard and understood. It also allows for clarification and promotes a verbal give-and-take. Common stems for summary paraphrasing include:

- "In other words, you're saying . . ."
- "Sounds like . . ."
- "What I'm hearing you say is . . ."

Summary paraphrasing requires more sophistication than restatement because the E-PFA sender must be accurate in their summary. While paraphrasing can clarify content and offer the receiver a new perspective, it is worth noting that paraphrases are essentially statements or closed-end questions. Someone experiencing low energy or difficulty processing information ("dumbing down") may respond with just a yes or no, without further elaboration. If this occurs, simply follow up with an open-ended question.

For example: "Sounds like you're feeling really sad? What does that feel like for you? What specific things are noticeable?"

Summary paraphrases can be used for both cognitive content and emotional content. In the case of emotional content, you would paraphrase the emotion expressed by the receiver. This emotion may be communicated directly through words, or it may be conveyed indirectly, through nonverbal displays. Paraphrases of emotional content might sound like:

- "You seem really upset."
- "Perhaps you're feeling angry."
- "You sound pretty depressed."
- "You look pretty confident."
- "Are you telling me you are really anxious right now?"

Paraphrases are effective tools for building empathy and rapport, demonstrating that the PFA provider is working hard to understand the person in distress. They encourage cathartic ventilation, instill hope, and clarify expressions, preventing potentially costly misunderstandings. Paraphrasing also validates emotions, which can help defuse an emotional spiral, regulate emotions, reduce confusion, and foster adherence to offered suggestions. For those experiencing momentary confusion (cortical inhibition), it may aid in identifying and accepting their emotions.

As mentioned previously, being aware of cultural and gender differences is important when reflecting emotions. In the United States, people are generally encouraged to be open about their feelings, whereas people from some non-American cultures may be more reserved (Pedersen et al., 2002). That said, men in the United States are often not socialized to express their feelings as openly as women (Cournoyer & Mahalik, 1995).

KEY POINTS

Let's briefly review the key points of this chapter, as well as other key points of Part One of the manual.

1) This chapter covers the basics of communication, emphasizing the importance of establishing rapport through nonverbal behavior, paralinguistic cues, and active listening techniques. Above all, it highlights the need to show up and convey a compassionate, supportive presence.

2) When actively listening, allow the receiver (person in distress) to tell their story—that is, what happened and what hurts. Encourage them to share only what they are comfortable revealing. Use paraphrases to make sure you correctly hear what they are saying, and to allow the receiver to hear their own thoughts and emotions. Remember to clarify words or phrases you do not understand, and ask "how bad" things are. Use questions, and observe nonverbal behavior to ascertain the severity of the distress and how much it interferes with daily life.

3) Use questions to determine the "worst part" of the situation and the receiver's reaction to it. Remember, close-ended questions can confirm, while open-ended questions can explore or probe.

4) Normalize their reactions, if appropriate. People in distress often feel their experiences are unique, but in reality their reactions are probably quite common given the circumstances. They should be reminded of that.

5) Provide reassurance, if appropriate. Try to foster an optimistic, hopeful vision, but do not make promises you cannot keep.

6) Foster resilience and self-empowerment through questions and direct statements. Most people in acute distress do not want

to be "rescued." They want assistance in helping themselves. Rushing to solve their problem, while sometimes necessary, can risk perpetuating the helplessness they may already feel.

7) Use questions like the following to help re-empower the person in distress and foster resilience:

"Can the problem be solved? If so, how?"

"Can the problem be buffered or mitigated? If so, how?"

"What can you do to reduce the intensity of the distress you are experiencing right now?"

"What things have helped you reduce stress in the past?"

"What can I do to help?"

8) Use statements to provide options: "Here are some things to think about and to try."

9) Use explanatory guidance by offering supportive, fact-based speculations in response to common questions like, "How did this happen?" "Why did this happen?" "Why me?" Avoid reinforcing any self-derogatory explanations the person may offer, such as, "I got what I deserve," "Bad things always happen to me," "I'm never lucky," "I will never be happy/successful." Stick to facts and compassionate reasoning.

10) Use anticipatory guidance to help shape expectations and prepare the person for what they might experience next. These statements can serve as gentle warnings based on common reactions to distress, such as, "You may have difficulty sleeping for a while." "You may find yourself feeling irritable." Ideally, these are based on the sender's own experiences or observations.

11) Use prescriptive guidance, offering suggestions or recommendations for coping and stress management. There are numerous effective stress-reduction and resilience-building strategies; see Everly & Lating (2019) for analysis and practical guidance.

12) If the level of distress is severe at the outset, does not begin to lessen, or seems to be increasing, consider encouraging the person to seek additional assistance, including professional mental health assessment and care.

References

Brammer, L. M., & MacDonald, G. (1996). *The helping relationship: Process and skills* (6th ed.). Allyn & Bacon.

Cournoyer, R. J., & Mahalik, J. R. (1995). Cross-sectional study of gender role conflict examining college-age and middle-aged men. *Journal of Counseling Psychology, 19*, 11–19. https://doi.org/10.1037/0022-0167.42.1.11

Everly, G. S., Jr., & Lating, J. M. (2019). *A clinical guide to the treatment of the human stress response* (4th ed.). Springer Science & Business Media.

Everly, G. S., Jr., & Mitchell, J. T. (2008). *Integrative crisis intervention and disaster mental health.* Chevron.

Ivey, A. E. (1994). *Intentional interviewing and counseling: Facilitating client development in a multicultural society* (3rd ed.). Brooks/Cole.

Mehrabian, A. (1971). *Silent messages.* Wadsworth.

Pedersen, P. B., Draguns, J. G., Lonner, W. J., & Trimble, J. E. (2002). *Counseling across cultures* (5th ed.). Sage.

PART II
EVERYDAY PSYCHOLOGICAL FIRST AID (E-PFA) FOR COMMON PSYCHOLOGICAL INJURIES AND CRISES

Just as a physical first aid manual offers guidance for assisting with physical injuries, this manual provides guidance for responding to psychological injuries and crises. Unlike physical first aid, however, the guidance offered here is not a form of treatment. It is intentionally less rigid and far more flexible, recognizing that no two people or situations are exactly alike. There is no cookie-cutter approach to E-PFA. Instead, this manual presents checklists of options to choose from, organized into five phases and 10 core questions. These tools are applied in the following 13 chapters, each addressing a different psychological condition. Some of these are presented in the context of diagnostic categories, while others reflect more common, nonclinical experiences.

Structure and Limitations

Each chapter in Part Two begins with a scenario that illustrates the psychological injury or crisis being addressed. This is followed by definitions, key features, and prevalence data. These descriptions often draw on the *Diagnostic and Statistical Manual of Mental Disorders* (5th ed., text rev.), commonly referred to as the *DSM-5-TR* (American Psychiatric Association, 2022), which provides standardized diagnostic criteria used by mental health professionals. We also frequently reference the World Health Organization (WHO), a United Nations agency focused on international public health.

After this descriptive material, each chapter offers optional guidance—referred to as potential E-PFA recommendations—on how the helper (i.e., the sender) in the scenario might apply the E-PFA model. While there is some overlap in the guidance across the 13 chapters, each chapter also reflects the unique aspects of the specific condition covered. Finally, each chapter concludes with a sample E-PFA dialogue, designed to demonstrate how the model can be applied in a natural, conversational way. The dialogues are intentionally flexible and loosely aligned with the recommended E-PFA options to reflect the adaptable nature of real-world interactions.

Every manual offering guidance of this kind has limitations. The optional recommendations in each chapter are general guidelines tailored to the specific topic. *They are not intended for verbatim application.* Ultimately, those applying E-PFA must combine their best judgment with the guidance provided here to help mitigate others' distress. If those efforts fall short, we recommend recruiting additional resources—either informally, such as friends and family, or formally, by calling 9-1-1 (local emergency services), 9-8-8 (National Suicide and Crisis Lifeline), primary care providers, psychological or psychiatric hotlines, or by helping the person access emergency services at a hospital or clinic.

With these caveats in mind, let's explore in detail some of the relevant psychological injuries and crises that may benefit from E-PFA.

BRENDAN IS 30 YEARS OLD. *Academically, he did very well in high school. He graduated with honors from a very highly regarded college and was immediately admitted to a top-ranked master of business administration (MBA) program, where he also excelled. After graduation, he was recruited to work at a successful and competitive finance firm. However, he encountered difficulties almost immediately after starting the job. The work was far more demanding than graduate school, and he was struggling. In addition, he was having trouble fitting in socially. About two weeks ago, he noticed a lack of energy but dismissed it as exhaustion from working 10- to 12-hour days. He has lost his appetite and sleeps poorly, awakening each night around three a.m. Though he used to go to the gym three days a week, he says he no longer has the time or energy. Someone at work approached him recently and asked why he always looks sad. Brendan agreed that he has been feeling depressed. Jake, Brendan's best friend since high school, typically speaks with him once or twice a week. Brendan reaches out to Jake, asking to talk about what's been going on. Jake, sensing Brendan's discomfort, agrees to stop by later that day after work.*

What Is Depression?

The term "depression" is often used in everyday conversation to describe a range of emotional states. It can mean different things to different people, so it's important to clarify what depression means to the person using the term.

The key feature of depression is a sad or depressed mood. It's fair to say that everyone has or will experience a passing case of sadness that may last several days, even up to a week. This sadness can be related to situational factors, such as change and uncertainty, loss, regret, or failure. It may also be related to a change in body physiology, such as physical exhaustion, low blood sugar, or even hormonal changes. When depression is temporary and not incapacitating, it's often called "the blues."

From the PFA perspective, both the transient situational blues and the more potentially incapacitating depression might be the focus of assistance. Interventions may start out much the same in both cases, but in the latter, we would be keenly aware of the need to help formulate a plan for accessing more advanced assistance.

Key Features: Signs and Symptoms

While not a comprehensive list, these are key signs and symptoms to look and listen for (American Psychiatric Association, 2022):

- Sad or depressed mood (melancholy) that in some cases may be accompanied with irritability
- Difficulty experiencing happiness, joy, or pleasure in things that typically bring pleasure (known as anhedonia)

- Lack of energy, chronic tiredness, reluctance or difficulty getting out of bed
- Psychomotor slowness or impairment in activities (e.g., walking)
- Difficulty sleeping (usually waking around two or three a.m.)
- Loss of appetite (though there may be an increase in consumption of "comfort foods")
- Loss of sex drive (decreased libido)
- Pervasive pessimism
- Helplessness, hopelessness
- Thoughts of death

Degrees of Depression

Rather than being strictly categorical, depression is thought to occur on a spectrum or continuum, meaning there is a wide variety of signs, symptoms, and severities (mild, moderate, severe). The greater the number of reactions listed below that the person acknowledges, and the greater their severity, the more urgent the need for attention and intervention.

Mild depression typically includes sadness, as well as difficulty being happy or optimistic. There is little or no interference with activities of daily life.

Moderate depression includes sadness and difficulty being happy or optimistic, combined with a general lack of energy, reluctance to get out of bed, and one or two other symptoms from the above checklist. There is typically mild to moderate interference with activities of daily life.

Severe depression usually encompasses a sad mood combined with several, if not most, of the symptoms listed above, resulting in significant or severe interference with fundamental life activities.

Prevalence of Depression

Depression is one of the most common forms of psychological distress. It affects people of all ages, races, and ethnicities. According to a Gallup poll in February 2023, 29% of Americans reported having been diagnosed with depression in their lifetime, and 17.8% reported currently experiencing depression. Not surprisingly, the overall prevalence of depression symptoms in the United States for adults was more than three times higher during COVID-19 compared to before the pandemic (Ettman et al., 2020). Adolescents appear uniquely vulnerable to depression due to the inherent developmental challenges of that age. According to the Centers for Disease Control and Prevention (2022), during the COVID-19 pandemic, 44% of US high school students reported persistent feelings of sadness or hopelessness, and only 47% reported feeling close to people at school.

Types of Depression

Not all depressions are alike. It can emerge in several recognizable patterns or syndromes, including the following:

Reactive Depression

Reactive (or situational) depression is the sudden emergence of depressive signs and symptoms in response to a highly stressful event or situation. In other words, some event or situation directly triggers the emergence of depressive symptoms. Most commonly, this type of depression resolves as the precipitating situation remits or is accepted. Symptoms can last anywhere from one or two weeks to several months, depending on the circumstances. It may be associated with the loss of a relationship, academic challenges, career setbacks, relocation (especially common among adolescents who are compelled to move at important developmental stages), or health-related challenges. For example, a study found that more than 27% of those recently unemployed reported reactive depressive symptoms (Perkonigg et al., 2018).

Persistent Depressive Disorder

Persistent depressive disorder (also known as dysthymia) is a chronic low-level depressed mood that lasts for most days over a period of at least two years and often seems unassociated with situational factors. According to the National Institute of Mental Health website (2024), the lifetime prevalence (percentage of people who will experience the syndrome over the course of a lifetime) is about 2.5%. A referral for professional assessment is often warranted.

Major Depression

Major depression is a constellation of the signs and symptoms listed above that lasts for more than two weeks and, most importantly, interferes with significant aspects of daily life. The lifetime prevalence of major depression varies based on the source, with estimates ranging from around 12%, according to the fifth edition of the *Diagnostic and Statistical Manual of Mental Disorders* (APA, 2022), to about 18.4% of the US population, according to a national study under the direction of the CDC (Lee et al., 2023). According to the World Health Organization (WHO, 2023) approximately 280 million people worldwide have depression. Medical and psychological assessments, as well as treatment referrals, are important in cases of major depression.

Seasonal Depression

Seasonal depression (also referred to as seasonal affective disorder or SAD) occurs in 1% to 10% of the population worldwide

(Meesters & Gordijn, 2016), with rates influenced by latitude, gender, age, and how it is measured. This form of depression is highly associated with seasonal change, especially winter.

Perinatal Depression

Perinatal depression includes depression that originates during pregnancy (prenatal depression) and depression that begins after the baby is born (postpartum depression). According to the WHO (2022), about 20% of women experience perinatal depression, which can last several months or more than a year. Medical and psychological assessments and treatments are important in these instances.

Potential E-PFA Recommendations
(Think About Trying This)

What can Brendan's friend Jake do to assist Brendan with his symptoms of depression? Listed below are potential E-PFA interventions that Jake might use. As noted, depression can be immobilizing and can erode self-esteem and self-confidence. Let's look at this situation through the five-step E-PFA model, expanded with the questions and options presented in italics:

1) Introduce yourself (if applicable), offer to help, set expectations, de-escalate (if needed).
2) Gather information. (*What happened? What hurts? How bad is it?*)
3) Clarify. (*What's the worst part?*)
4) Provide assistance. (*What do you need right now? How can I help?*)
   a. *Can Jake use problem-focused assistance?*
   b. *Can Jake use emotion-focused assistance?*
   c. *Can Jake use stress management?*
5) Make a plan. (*Next steps?*)

Introduce Yourself, Offer to Help, Set Expectations, De-escalate

- If possible, Jake should physically meet with Brendan. He could use a virtual platform like Zoom or FaceTime if in-person contact is not possible. Showing up to assist reduces the sense of isolation and shows the person that somebody cares. In this scenario, Jake shows up in person to meet with Brendan.
- PFA begins with Jake showing up, expressing concern, and letting Brendan know he wants to help. And if he can't help, he will assist Brendan in finding the help he needs. No introduction is necessary because they know each other.

Gather Information

- Encourage the process of verbal venting or catharsis. Jake should allow Brendan to talk about his work and what he is experiencing. Questions like "What's going on?" or "Tell me what's happening at work" can begin the conversation. (*What happened?*)
- Once Brendan describes the details of his work situation, Jake can ask how the problems are affecting his life. For example, "That sounds really tough. How are the problems at work impacting you? How are they showing up in your daily life?" (*What hurts?*)
- Even though Brendan will have described the daily impacts, Jake can ask about their overall severity. For example, "So how big a problem is this?" Or, "This sounds really distressing. How bad is it? How much is it disrupting your life?" (*How bad is it?*)

Clarify

- The clarification phase might begin with Jake paraphrasing or recapping what he has heard. For example, "I'm really sorry about all that's going on. It sounds like this job hasn't worked out so far as you had hoped. Sounds like graduate school didn't necessarily prepare you for the 'real world' the way you thought it would. I can see why you sound kind of depressed. It must be really frustrating."

- After the summary paraphrase, Jake can ask a follow-up question: "So what's the worst part of this for you?" He should listen carefully to Brendan's answer because it will give him some idea of where to start to assist beyond the active listening he's already done. (*What's the worst part?*)

Provide Assistance

- Before making specific suggestions, Jake might ask, "What do you need right now?" or "How can I help?" These questions can guide him to the next possible steps. Another helpful question might be "What has helped you cope in the past?" If this approach fails to help, Jake might adopt a more directive approach by using suggestions from one or more of the active ingredients listed below. If Jake is unsure where to begin, Brendan's response to the question about "the worst part" might help him decide.

Problem-Focused

- It would be natural for Brendan to think he should quit his job. While that might be a solution, it's probably too soon to make that decision. It's important for Jake to discourage Brendan from making any significant life changes without thorough thought and consultation with someone who can be objective.
- Jake can talk with Brendan about the possibility of discussing his challenges with his supervisor.
- He can also discuss the possibility of Brendan getting tutorial or mentoring support.

Emotion-Focused

- Jake could assist Brendan change his perspective on these work challenges. Brendan feels like a failure. He expected to learn the job quickly and excel. Were these appropriate assumptions? Jake can help Brendan see that his expectations for immediate success might not have been realistic.
- Brendan might think he is the only person who has ever encountered this situation. Jake can encourage him to talk to others at work to see if anyone else has experienced similar reactions when they first started.
- Rather than blame the job or Brendan's graduate school, Jake can empower Brendan by asking whether he can see himself taking responsibility for improving his own performance.
- Jake could ask Brendan what Brendan might say to Jake if their situations were reversed (role reversal).

Stress Management-Focused

- Jake can encourage Brendan to resume regular visits to the gym. Physical exercise has been shown to improve mood and self-confidence, and it is something Brendan mentioned he used to enjoy.
- Jake can encourage Brendan to get out of his apartment, even if it's just to take a walk.
- He can also remind Brendan that early mornings (due to tiredness) and late nights (due to darkness and isolation) are likely to be the most difficult times of day for him.

Make a Plan

If it doesn't get scheduled, it doesn't get done. Because Jake knows Brendan, follow-up seems reasonable.

- If possible, every E-PFA intervention should end by making a plan for next steps. This is true even if this is the first and only contact Jake will have with Brendan. Jake can ask Brendan what he plans to do to help himself. "So, Brendan, let's talk about next steps. Let's make a plan for moving beyond this situation." Jake can also ask Brendan to write the plan down and send it to him.

- Jake can encourage Brendan to talk to other friends and family.
- He can ask Brendan to discuss his depressive symptoms with Brendan's primary care provider if they persist or worsen.
- When possible, Jake should follow up with Brendan to see how he is doing and ask if he has sought further support.

E-PFA Dialogue (It Might Sound Like This)

Here is an example of a brief E-PFA intervention if Jake stopped by Brendan's apartment after work. While each conversation will differ, the following dialogue incorporates some of the recommendations from the previous section. This will serve as a model for the dialogues in the remaining chapters.

BRENDAN: Hi Jake. Good to see you. Thanks for taking the time to meet with me today. I shared with you over text that I'm struggling, so I'm really glad you were able to stop by so soon.

JAKE: Of course. I don't know what's happening, but it's usually good to talk during difficult times. I'll do all I can to help, and that starts with listening. If I think you need more help than I'm capable of offering, I'll assist with that too. Sound good?

BRENDAN: Sounds good. Thanks.

JAKE: So, what's going on?

BRENDAN: I don't know exactly what it is, but something's wrong . . . and it's clearly impacting my work.

JAKE: Tell me what's happening at work.

BRENDAN: The job is much tougher than I expected. I'm having trouble meeting deadlines, and my supervisor recently assigned me to work with someone else on one of my projects. I'm having difficulty concentrating at work, and to be honest, Jake, it's hard right now for me to even care. I just kind of feel down all the time.

JAKE: That sounds really tough, Brendan. How are the problems at work impacting you? I mean, how are they showing up in your daily life? In other words, what hurts?

BRENDAN: What hurts is an interesting question, Jake. I might describe it as a painful numbness, where I can't seem to find pleasure in much of anything for the past several weeks. And even though I'm exhausted when I go to bed at night, I'm waking up around two or three a.m. most mornings, and when I do, it's miserable. It often takes me an hour to fall back asleep, and then when the alarm sounds, I don't want to get out of bed. When I do finally get out of bed, I feel like I'm moving in slow motion . . . and this continues during most of my workday. You know how much I enjoy going to the gym. Well, I haven't been in two weeks.

JAKE: This sounds really distressing, Brendan. How bad is it?

BRENDAN: I'm thinking this job is way too much for me. I'm in over my head and I don't feel prepared or capable. Oh, and listen to this—I had a coworker approach me two days ago, and she said I looked depressed. Can you see now why I called you?

JAKE: I'm really sorry this job hasn't worked out as you hoped so far. Sounds like graduate school didn't necessarily prepare you for the "real world" as much as you had thought it would. I can see why you sound kind of down or even depressed.

Maybe your coworker is right? You're feeling sad, you're not sleeping, you're not finding any pleasure in much of anything, and you're not exercising. It sounds like you have symptoms of depression, which I certainly can tell aren't comfortable.

BRENDAN: I think you're right, Jake.

JAKE: What's the worst part for you?

BRENDAN (PAUSE): I feel like I've lost my edge.

JAKE: When you say, "lost my edge," what do you mean?

BRENDAN: I'm just not myself. I don't feel confident.

JAKE: How can I help?

BRENDAN: I don't think there is anything you can do.

JAKE: What has helped you cope in the past when you've had problems or challenges?

BRENDAN: I tough them out, but this is different. In fact, I'm thinking I should quit the job.

JAKE: I can understand why you would think about quitting, because it might solve the immediate problem. However, given what you're currently going through, now is not the best time to make big, life-altering decisions. You should give this some serious thought before considering it. And maybe talk with someone who is more objective?

BRENDAN: Like who?

JAKE: How do you get along with your supervisor?

BRENDAN (PAUSE): She's very approachable.

JAKE: You may not feel comfortable reaching out to her, but if she's as approachable as you say, it might be worth considering the risk of talking with her about what you're experiencing. Maybe she can help by connecting you with someone more experienced who can serve as a mentor or tutor. Who knows, maybe that's why she's having someone else work with you on one of your projects.

BRENDAN: I see what you're saying, but I just don't want to appear weak or incompetent. I thought for sure I'd excel at this job. I don't want to fail.

JAKE: You've been accustomed to success since I've known you in high school. And I'm sure that with time, you'll succeed professionally as well. However, you went directly from the security of graduate school to working at a major finance firm. To borrow a baseball analogy, you've gone from the minors to the big leagues without a lot of game experience. I imagine that, just like in baseball, very few succeed in this environment right away. In fact, you might want to chat with some of your colleagues about how they adjusted to the world of big-time finance. And while it's certainly possible that some of your challenges are due to gaps in your graduate school training or the job expectations, right now you're trying to succeed when you're not at your physical or emotional best. Let's talk about what we can do to work on that.

BRENDAN: I hear what you're saying, Jake, and I appreciate the perspective and encouragement. I need to give this some more time to get better.

JAKE: Let me ask you this: What would you say to me if the situation were reversed, and I was the one struggling?

BRENDAN: Likely, pretty much the same thing, and I'd add that it's important to get back to the gym.

JAKE: Good call, Brendan! Exercising improves mood and self-confidence, and you enjoy it. Even if you don't go to the gym daily, you should get out of your apartment to take a walk. As you're hopefully considering these suggestions, keep in mind that mornings and late nights might be the most difficult parts of your day. Something you could try is drinking water as soon as you wake up. It keeps you hydrated, fuels your brain, and helps with digestion and metabolism. And make sure you eat healthily and regularly during the day.

BRENDAN: This is all very helpful Jake.

JAKE: So, let's talk about next steps or a plan to help you move beyond this situation. It will be helpful to write down what we've talked about and send it to me, if you're okay with that.

BRENDAN: That sounds good. We've covered a lot. Writing it down will help me to remember and follow through.

JAKE: I'm glad we had this conversation, but I also encourage you to talk with other family and friends you feel comfortable with.

BRENDAN: That's a good idea. But I'm relieved I started with you. I'm feeling more positive and hopeful.

JAKE: That's good to hear, Brendan. If the depressive symptoms you've described get worse or don't start to improve, reach out to your primary care physician for more help.

BRENDAN: I understand. And that makes sense. And I will.

JAKE: Listen, I'm not going away. It might take some time, maybe even a week or so, for you to start feeling like yourself again and get back into your routine. How about you and I touch base in a few days to talk about how your plan is going and any possible next steps?

BRENDAN: Thanks, Jake. I look forward to it.

References

American Psychiatric Association. (2022). Depressive disorders. In *Diagnostic and statistical manual of mental disorders* (5th ed., text rev.). https://doi.org/10.1176/appi.books.9780890425787.x04_Depressive Disorders

Centers for Disease Control and Prevention. (2022). *New CDC data illuminate youth mental health threats during the COVID-19 pandemic.* https://www/cdc.gov/media/releases/2022/p0331-youth-mental -health-covid-19.html

Ettman, C. K., Abdalla, S. M., Cohen, G. H., Sampson, L., Vivier, P. M., & Galea, S. (2020). Prevalence of depression symptoms in US adults before and during the COVID-19 pandemic. *JAMA Network Open,* 3(9): e2019686. https://doi.org/10.1001/jamanetworkopen.2020 .19686

Gallup. (2023, May). *U.S. depression rates reach new highs.* https://news .gallup.com/poll/505745/depression-rates-reach-new-highs.aspx

Lee, B., Wang, Y., Carlson, S. A., Greenlund, K. J., Lu, H., Liu, Y., Croft, J. B., Eke, P. I., Town, M., & Thomas, C. W. (2023). National, state-level, and county-level prevalence estimates of adults aged ≥ 18 years self-reporting a lifetime diagnosis of depression—United States, 2020. *CDC: Morbidity and Mortality Weekly Report,* 72(24), 644–650.

Meesters, Y., & Gordijn, M. C. M. (2016). Seasonal affective disorder, winter type: Current insights and treatment options. *Psychology Research and Behavior Management,* 9, 317–327. https://doi.org/10.2147 /PRBM.S114906

National Institute of Mental Health. (2024). *Persistent depressive disorder (dysthymic disorder).* https://www.nimh.nih.gov/health /statistics/persistent-depressive-disorder-dysthymic-disorder

Perkonigg, A., Lorenz, L., & Maercker, A. (2018). Prevalence and correlates of ICD-11 adjustment disorder: Findings from the Zurich Adjustment Disorder Study. *International Journal of Clinical and Health Psychology,* 18(3), 209–217. https://doi.org/10.1016/j.ijchp.2018 .05.001

World Health Organization. (2022). *WHO guide for integration of perinatal mental health in maternal and child health services.* https:// www.who.int/publications/i/item/9789240057142

World Health Organization. (2023). *Depressive disorder (depression).* https://www.who.int/news-room/fact-sheets/detail/depression

SIX | Stress

IT'S 9:05 A.M. *on a frigid Thursday morning in February, and 44-year-old Keenan is 35 minutes late for work. When he arrives, his coworker Clayton notices that Keenan is disheveled, his hands are dirty, and he appears frazzled. Without Clayton saying or asking anything, Keenan explains that it's been quite the past 18 hours. He begins by noting the email that everyone in the company received the day before stating that there would be no cost-of-living or merit increase in salaries this year. Keenan tells Clayton that before he could tell his wife about this unfortunate news, she informed him that she was being laid off from her factory job in two weeks. His wife also said that her parents, who had been staying with them for a week and were supposed to leave on Friday, and with whom Keenan has a lukewarm relationship at best, were going to be staying with them for at least several more weeks. Keenan tells Clayton that he went to bed early but had a tough time sleeping. He notes that as he was showering this morning, the stall, which he paid to have fixed six months ago, was leaking. As he was driving to work, he ran*

into a pothole that flattened the front passenger-side tire of his car.
Keenan pulled over and changed the tire before arriving at work. Keenan
says, "That's been my past day." What does Clayton say?

What Is Stress?

In his groundbreaking book *The Stress of Life*, Hans Selye (1956) makes two critical assertions: (1) stress is the response of the mind and body to any demand placed on them, and (2) the absence of stress is death. Stress is a physical and psychological, or mind-body, reaction to life experiences (Girdano et al., 2013). Simply put, stress is a part of life!

Stress is related to and even underlies anxiety (see Chapter Eight), fear (see Chapter Seven), and traumatic stress (see Chapter Eleven). It is the main driver, physiologically speaking, of all these conditions. Stress has positive and negative aspects. Before discussing its more harmful, and notable, effects, it's important to note that stress is not always detrimental. In fact, there is what is known as "eustress," or good stress, a certain amount of which can help increase focus and attention and lead to optimal performance. This means stress can serve as a positive, motivating form of arousal. Getting "psyched up" for an event is an example.

Furthermore, stress, like fear, is a natural physical response that accelerates the body's defenses when threatened. The stress response was crucial in prehistoric times, when we were more frequently exposed to life-threatening emergencies (e.g., being attacked by predators). It evolved as a survival mechanism. Today, however, stress can often become overwhelming, fatiguing, and can impair daily activities or even lead to illness.

When trying to understand the nature of human stress (or anxiety, fear, and panic), it is important to realize that most stress in our lives stems from how we perceive and interpret ourselves, other people, and our environment. Hans Selye, though he studied the biology of human stress, ultimately concluded, "It's not what happens to you that matters, it's how you take it." This notion, borrowed from the Stoic philosophers of ancient Greece, asserts that we are disturbed not by events, but by our views and interpretations of those events. This is a critical claim, because although we cannot always control what happens to us, we can control how we react. Exceptions to this rule include stress caused by physical injury, pain, hormonal imbalances, and drugs. In general, however, the good news is that most human stress is self-created and can be greatly reduced by altering our reactions. This is especially relevant in the current age of social media, where the endless pursuit of "likes" and the rise of cyberbullying contribute to stress.

Key Features: Signs and Symptoms

Psychology of the Stress Response

Change your attitude, change your world! This idea emphasizes that stress, like beauty, resides in the eye of the beholder. See the figures below, which are derived from information contained in Chapter Three and underscore this point. The first figure shows that stressful events, called stressors, set the stage for a stress response but do not cause it. The second figure shows that by altering one's attitude, interpretation, and overall appraisal of situations,

Interpretation and Stress

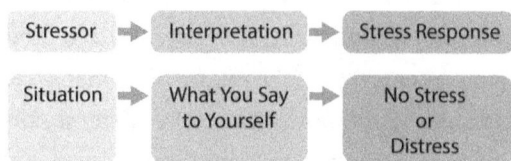

Stressor ➡ Interpretation ➡ Stress Response

Situation ➡ What You Say to Yourself ➡ No Stress or Distress

Changing Interpretation and Stress

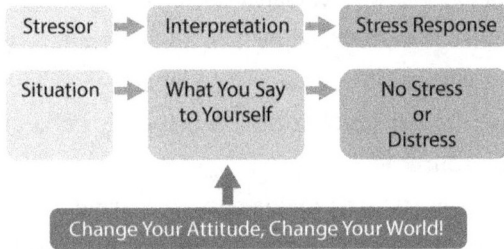

Stressor	➡	Interpretation	➡	Stress Response
Situation	➡	What You Say to Yourself	➡	No Stress or Distress

⬆

Change Your Attitude, Change Your World!

it is possible to mitigate or even prevent excessive stress, called "distress" in the E-PFA model.

Biology of the Stress Response

Walter Cannon—a Harvard physiologist, Nobel laureate, and pioneer in the study of stress—was interested in how the body maintains balance, or a "steady state." He described stress as the "fight-or-flight" response (1939), a term now familiar to most. Cannon theorized that when a person perceives a threat, the brain quickly assesses the situation and triggers a cascade of neurochemicals that prepare the body to act in ways to lessen the risk. This invaluable hardwired alarm system is meant to mobilize the body's resources quickly and efficiently. The acute, survival-oriented stress response includes several key psychophysiological reactions, such as:

- Increased blood pressure and heart rate (to help circulate more blood and oxygen)
- Increased breathing rate (to increase oxygen supply, which helps the brain and muscles respond)
- Pupils dilate (to enable you to see more of the possible threat)
- Airways in lungs dilate (to enable you to breathe in more oxygen to help the circulation process)

- Hearing becomes more attuned (to make you more alert)
- Skin gets cold and sweaty: Warm blood is diverted from the surface of the skin to reduce bleeding if injured. Sweating, triggered by increased glucose, makes you more slippery—and harder to catch
- Digestive system shuts down (digestion is not a good use of needed resources)
- Glucose levels rise (to provide needed energy)
- Muscles tense (in preparation for fighting or fleeing)
- Memory is enhanced

The immediate human stress response is a well-orchestrated combination of physical and chemical reactions that help manage short-term threats to well-being—and are essentially the same for all individuals. One key chemical released during the stress response is the hormone adrenaline, which comes from the adrenal medulla, the inner part of the adrenal glands, located atop the kidneys. In moderate amounts, adrenaline acts as a supercharger, boosting strength, endurance, and even learning (see Everly & Lating, 2019, for a comprehensive review). Notably, adrenaline levels rise with the ingestion of energy drinks.

Cortisol is another hormone involved in the stress response. After the hypothalamus—the part of the brain that triggers the stress response—sends signals to the pituitary gland, the pituitary releases a hormone that in turn signals the adrenal cortices (outer layers of the adrenal glands) to increase cortisol production. Cortisol is naturally produced at varying levels throughout the day, but during a stressful event, its levels rise sharply. This surge increases the availability of energy (including a tenfold increase in glucose), activates the immune system as needed, and reduces inflammation (McEwen, 2019). Once the acute threat is over—say, the predator is gone—the stress response, including the release of adrenaline and cortisol, is designed to subside, allowing the body to return to its prethreat state.

Prevalence of Excessive Stress

To provide additional context, here are some findings on the effects of various stressors:

- In a 2022 survey of adults from 142 countries, 40% reported experiencing high levels of stress (Gallup, 2023).
- The American Psychological Association's Stress in America study (2023) reported that health-related stressors (65%), the economy (64%), and money (63%) were the top sources of stress among adults surveyed, with women reporting higher stress levels than men.
- A large study on reasons for primary care physician visits showed an increase in visits related to anxiety and stress—from 29.9% in 2006–2007 to 38.0% in 2014–2015—then a slight decrease to 34.5% in 2018, just before COVID (Rosenstein et al., 2023).
- The COVID-19 pandemic had a profound impact on mental health, including stress. In a global study of 26 countries using a standardized stress questionnaire (scoring from 0 to 40, with a historical average of 13.1), scores ranged from near average in Switzerland (13.3) to 21.7 in Turkey and 17.5 in the United States—both Turkey and the United States showing significantly higher scores than the normal average (Kowal et al., 2020).
- In a global study of hospital staff treating COVID-19 patients, 45% reported experiencing excessive stress (Salari et al., 2020).

Functional Categories of Stress Reactions

The previous section discussed the stress response as an acute survival mechanism intended to be activated for short periods of time. But stress actually falls into three functional categories: (1) eustress (positive, motivating stress that helps you survive and achieve), (2) distress (short-term excitation that is uncomfortable and distracting), and (3) dysfunction/impairment (excessive stress that is either too intense or too prolonged, interfering with daily life and the ability to accomplish important tasks). Listed below are some, but not all, signs and symptoms of two of these categories, further broken down by how they manifest. Eustress is not reviewed here, as its signs and symptoms largely overlap with those listed above. Instead, let's focus on stress when it fails to be helpful.

Cognitive (Thinking)

Distress

These are temporary in duration, and mild to moderate in intensity.

- Temporary confusion, time distortion
- Difficulty concentrating
- Reduced problem-solving abilities (known as cortical inhibition)
- Repetitive thoughts (obsessions) about the distressing event
- Reliving or replaying the event
- Difficulty prioritizing

Dysfunction

These may be temporary or longer-lasting, interfering with life.

- Memory lapses
- Incapacitating confusion, diminished ability to think clearly and solve problems
- Hopelessness (see Chapter Five)
- Suicidal/homicidal thoughts (see Chapter Sixteen)
- Delusions (e.g., paranoid; see Chapter Seventeen)
- Hallucinations (see Chapter Seventeen)

- Evidence of an out-of-body or dissociative experience (not due to psychosis)

Emotional
Distress
These are temporary in duration, mild to moderate in intensity.

- Guilt (see Chapter Fourteen)
- Numbness
- Repeated procrastination
- Fear (see Chapter Seven)
- Sadness (see Chapter Five)
- Anger (see Chapter Nine)
- Irritability
- Mood swings
- Grief (see Chapter Fifteen)
- Anxiety (see Chapter Eight)

Dysfunction
These may be temporary or longer-lasting, interfering with life.

- Panic attacks (see Chapter Ten)
- Immobilizing depression, grief, or guilt (see Chapters Five, Fifteen, and Fourteen)
- Extreme emotional numbing
- Acute or posttraumatic stress disorder (PTSD; see Chapter Eleven)

Behavioral
Distress
These are temporary in duration, mild to moderate in intensity.

- Crying
- Withdrawn/reserved

- Sleep disturbances (e.g., falling or staying asleep)
- Excessive eating, especially comfort foods (see Chapter Twelve)
- Easily startled
- Temporary avoidance of places or people that bring back reminders of an upsetting event
- Compulsions (repetitive behaviors that are intended to alleviate anxiety by providing a sense of safety)
- Hoarding
- Hypervigilance
- Diminished personal hygiene
- Excessive use of energy supplements

Dysfunction

These may be temporary or longer-lasting, interfering with life.

- Alcohol/drug use to self-medicate, including prescription medications (see Chapter Thirteen)
- Recurrent 1,000-yard stare and unresponsiveness
- Persistent avoidance
- Impulsiveness, risk-taking
- Aggression, violence (see Chapter Nine)
- Immobilizing compulsions
- Immobility
- Self-isolation
- Missing work
- Lack of personal hygiene
- Extreme insomnia

Physical

Distress

These are temporary in duration, mild to moderate in intensity. *Note:* Any prolonged occurrence (lasting more than a couple of days) of physical changes or other symptoms of concern should be evaluated by a medical professional.

- Headaches
- Hyperventilation
- Muscle cramps, aches, or spasms
- Fatigue or exhaustion
- Disturbances in eating (see Chapter Twelve)
- Nausea

Dysfunction

These may be temporary or longer-lasting, interfering with life. *Note:* Seek medical attention for any of the following symptoms.

- Chest pain
- Persistent irregular heartbeats
- Dizziness
- Loss of consciousness
- Any type of apparent seizure
- Blood in stool or urine
- Numbness or paralysis (e.g., arm, leg, or face)
- Inability to talk or understand speech

Spiritual

Distress

These are temporary in duration, mild to moderate in intensity.

- Anger at God (in whatever form that might be)
- Crisis of faith

Dysfunction

These may be temporary or longer-lasting, interfering with life.

- Discontinuation of one's faith practice

- Withdrawal from one's faith community
- Religious hallucinations or delusions

Notes on Reactions

As emphasized in Chapters Two and Three, it is important to consider each person individually when evaluating presenting signs and symptoms, the degree of functional impairment, and interference with activities of daily life (Everly & Lating, 2022). It's equally important not to assume that someone has a disorder or requires additional care solely based on the presence of *some* symptoms, particularly signs of distress. At the same time, symptoms indicative of dysfunction should not be minimized or overlooked, and appropriate care should be provided when needed.

Chronic Stress

The body, as described above, is designed to handle short-term stress. Unfortunately, it is far less effective at coping with repeated, prolonged, or chronic stress (Hussenoeder et al., 2022). Short-term physical stressors (e.g., changing a tire in extremely cold weather) require an immediate response, are temporary, and dissipate once action is taken. The body is well equipped to handle such situations. In contrast, most modern stressors stem from our psychological perceptions or interpretations of ongoing life events (e.g., relationships, finances, work, school). These are known as psychosocial stressors, and they usually cannot be quickly resolved through a simple physical response.

From a chronic stress perspective, once a stressor gets past our psychological defenses—that is, once it is interpreted as stressful—the body prepares for action (Girdano, et al., 2013). As noted, psychosocial stressors are virtually endless, and they affect people differently depending on genetic, social, spiritual, and environmental factors. The result is a stress response that is activated with a frequency, intensity, and, most detrimentally, a duration it simply wasn't intended to sustain.

Allostatic Load

Chronic, lifelong exposure to psychosocial stressors can disrupt the body's physiological regulatory systems responsible for initiating, maintaining, and shutting down the stress response, leading to increased wear and tear on the body and greater susceptibility to disease (Seeman et al., 2001). This repeated activation of the stress response—without sufficient time to recover, and requiring ongoing internal physiological adjustments—is known as "allostatic load" (McEwen, 1998; McEwen & Wingfield, 2003). One example of this wear and tear is the prolonged elevation of the stress hormone cortisol, which can contribute to weight gain (often in the abdomen), hypertension, reduced bone density, hyperglycemia (high blood sugar), muscle weakness, mood disturbances, and compromised immune function.

Burnout

The physiological changes and potential damage caused by allostatic load can lead to burnout. Herbert Freudenberger, a German-born American psychologist who coined the term in the 1970s, described burnout as "a depletion or exhaustion of a person's mental and physical resources attributed to his or her prolonged, yet unsuccessful striving toward unrealistic expectations, internally or externally derived" (1984, p. 223). While most commonly, and clinically, associated with occupational stress (World Health Organization, 2019), burnout is not considered a formal medical condition. It is, however, now broadly recognized as a state of emotional, mental, and physical exhaustion characterized by fatigue, apathy, lack of motivation, lack of empathy, dissatisfaction with work or other aspects of life, and other signs of personal distress, such as sleep difficulties, headaches, and changes in eating habits. When someone is burned out, their life balance is out of alignment, and they may become too exhausted to function effectively.

Although burnout has been a part of the vernacular for almost 50 years, its effects were heightened and highlighted during the COVID-19 pandemic, particularly among health care professionals. In a global study of 32,724 health care workers, 52% reported burnout and 51% reported emotional exhaustion during the pandemic (Ghahramani et al., 2021).

General Adaptation Syndrome

Nearly 70 years ago, Hans Selye introduced the concept of general adaptation syndrome (GAS) to describe the progression of the human stress response (1956). His GAS model consisted of three stages:

- The *alarm stage*, when the body exhibits a general, widespread arousal in response to stress (as described above)
- The *resistance stage*, when the body mobilizes physical, emotional, and behavioral resources to adapt and attempt to combat the stressor
- The *exhaustion stage*, when prolonged activation of the stress response can lead to disease, malfunction of organ systems, or even death

Here are some examples of physical and psychological disorders associated with the exhaustion phase:

- Muscle tension in the head, neck, and shoulders, which has been shown to be associated with tension and migraine headaches (Schramm et al., 2015)
- Low back pain (Choi et al., 2021)
- Chronic obstructive pulmonary disease (COPD; Lu et al., 2012)

- Increased risk of hypertension (Liu et al., 2017) and atherosclerosis (Gao et al., 2022)
- In children, increased risk of asthma attacks (Sandberg et al., 2000)
- Gastrointestinal diseases, resulting from the interconnected pathways between the brain and the gut, known as the gut-brain axis (Labanski et al., 2020)
- Changes in the diet, linked to obesity (Bremner et al., 2020)
- Diabetes (Sharma & Singh, 2020)
- Posttraumatic stress disorder (PTSD; see Chapter Eleven)

One classic example of the association between stress and PTSD describes the effects on those living within five miles (eight km) of the Three Mile Island nuclear power plant in Pennsylvania, which was involved in the release of radiation in 1979 (Davidson & Baum, 1986). More recently, chronic stress has been associated with PTSD symptoms in children (Kim et al., 2022).

Potential E-PFA Recommendations
(Think About Trying This)

What should Clayton say to Keenan? What would you say if you were in a position similar to Clayton's? This is clearly a case where stress management can play an important role in helping Clayton.

Let's look at this situation through the five-step E-PFA intervention, expanded with the questions and options presented in italics:

1) Introduce yourself (if applicable), offer to help, set expectations, de-escalate (if needed).
2) Gather information. (*What happened? What hurts? How bad is it?*)
3) Clarify. (*What's the worst part?*)

4) Provide assistance. (*What do you need right now? How can I help?*)

   a. *Can Clayton use problem-focused assistance?*

   b. *Can Clayton use emotion-focused assistance?*

   c. *Can Clayton use stress management?*

5) Make a plan. (*Next steps?*)

Introduce Yourself, Offer to Help, Set Expectations, De-escalate

- In this instance of acute distress, the first step for Clayton might be to help lower the stress Keenan is experiencing in the moment. Therefore, it is important for Clayton to present himself in a calm, supportive manner.

- Given that Keenan looks "frazzled," Clayton might employ de-escalation tactics. Clayton should speak a bit more slowly than usual and try to appear relaxed. He could suggest that Clayton follow him to a quiet place where they can talk. He might even suggest taking a couple of diaphragmatic breaths together.

Gather Information

- In this scenario Keenan has already vented and described the multiple sources of his distress. (*What happened?*) But he hasn't described how he is feeling about them. Clayton can ask Keenan how the stress is showing up for him. (*What hurts?*)

- Once Keenan describes how he is feeling, Clayton can try to gauge the severity of the stress response (how impairing it is) and determine if Keenan's reactions pose a serious threat to his well-being or the well-being of others. Remember, severity is defined as the interaction of intensity, urgency, and duration. (*How bad is it?*)

Clarify

- Here, Clayton's use of paraphrasing may be especially useful given the perfect storm Keenan has been experiencing.

- Clayton asking Keenan what the worst part of the situation is might help Keenan focus and feel less overwhelmed.

Provide Assistance

- Clayton can ask Keenan something like, "What do you need right now?" or "How can I help?" If this approach fails to help, Clayton can offer more direct assistance, as described next. If Clayton is unsure where to begin, Keenan's response to the question about "the worst part" might help him decide.

Problem-Focused

- Clayton might use a problem-solving or problem-mitigation approach, even if it lacks specific details, to help Keenan begin to feel more in control. Asking Keenan if he has any thoughts on problem-solving, or whether some assistance with it might help, is a reasonable place to start.

Emotion-Focused

- Clayton acknowledging or pointing out that Keenan seems to be feeling out of control transforms the intangible sense of being overwhelmed into something more tangible—and therefore more manageable.
- Clayton observing that Keenan seems to be surrendering his well-being to people and things outside his control may help Keenan focus on the one thing he can control: himself.
- Clayton can remind Keenan that, as Hans Selye, the father of stress concepts, once said, "It's not what happens to you that matters, it's how you take it." This perspective can be an important step in resilience and empowerment.

Stress Management–Focused

Stress management incorporates a range of physical and psychological strategies aimed at preventing or building resistance to stressors (e.g., changing one's environment to reduce exposure) or lessening their impact when exposure does occur. Effective stress management begins with recognizing what triggers stress and making good decisions to relieve its effects. Physical practices like exercise, meditation, and yoga are widely used to alleviate stress and promote relaxation (Edwards & Loprinzi, 2017; Sharma, 2014). However, because modern stress is often rooted in our perceptions and interpretations, it is imperative to understand how our thoughts shape our stress responses. Developing this awareness—and having a basic understanding of the stress response—can help us manage its adverse effects. This is where PFA can be so helpful.

- Clayton can start by asking Keenan how he has coped with stress in the past.
- He can ask Keenan what helps him feel relaxed, safe, and comfortable.
- He can ask what Keenan would say to Clayton if their situations were reversed.

These pointers can help Keenan begin the process of regaining a sense of control.

Make a Plan

- Clayton can help Keenan identify practical steps to reduce stress and regain a sense of control. While addressing all of Keenan's concerns may require more than one meeting, choosing one tangible action he can take now, tonight, or tomorrow would be a useful starting point. (*Where do we go from here? What are the next steps?*)

E-PFA Dialogue (It Might Sound Like This)

CLAYTON (PROJECTING A CALM, SUPPORTIVE PRESENCE):
Wow! It seems like you've been put through the wringer,
Keenan. Why don't we go to the break room so you can
decompress and we can talk?

KEENAN: Thanks Clayton, but I'm already late. I don't want to
make incredibly stressful matters even worse.

CLAYTON: I understand, but this is important. Besides, the 10
a.m. meeting got pushed back until noon, so there's no rush to
get there. So, come on. Let's go sit in the break room.

(They walk into the break room, which Clayton had already confirmed
was empty.)

CLAYTON: Let me grab you a water while you get comfortable.

(Clayton hands Keenan the water bottle and sits across from him. Both
are in reasonably comfortable chairs.)

CLAYTON: My wife and I have been going to a yoga class twice a
week for the past three months, and a basic part of the class is
using your breathing to help you feel centered and relaxed. It
really works. Do you mind if I show you how to do it? You
certainly seem like you could use it.

KEENAN: Right now, I'll take any help.

CLAYTON: Okay, so it's in through the nose, and slowly out
through the mouth.

KEENAN (TAKING A FEW DEEP BREATHES): I need this.

CLAYTON: For what it's worth, it helps no matter how you're
feeling. But it seems that so much has stacked up on you
in the past 18 hours. How is the stress showing up
for you?

KEENAN: I feel like I've been hit with a sledgehammer. My insides were racing last night and again this morning. I couldn't think straight, and I have very little appetite. Even though I felt fatigued, I had trouble getting to sleep because my mind kept racing. The last thing I needed was the flat tire on the way in this morning. I'm just not sure if I'm going to make it. It just seems like too much.

CLAYTON: I appreciate you sharing this with me. And again, your plate is more than full. A couple of things you just said caught my attention. The first being that you felt like your insides were racing.

KEENAN: Yeah, but this feels a little better now. The breathing and the water seem to be helping me to slightly settle down.

CLAYTON: Okay, that's good. Keep drinking the water and relaxing. Did you also experience any chest pains or feel like your heart wasn't beating right?

KEENAN: No . . . no, I didn't.

CLAYTON: Although the symptoms that you describe certainly aren't comfortable, they're not unexpected. I'd be more concerned if you were having signs of heart issues. The other thing you said was that you felt this was all too much and that you weren't going to make it. What do you mean by that?

KEENAN: I was just expressing how unexpected and oppressive this all feels. It's a lot.

CLAYTON: I'd regret if I didn't ask you to clarify, Keenan. Should I be concerned about your well-being or you possibly thinking of hurting or killing yourself?

KEENAN: I'll admit when my mind was racing a bit last night, there was a fleeting thought that I might be better off dead . . . but that was it! It came and rapidly went. I have too much to live for. So, no . . . no possible way I'd ever hurt myself—or anyone else. *(Starting to chuckle.)* Including my in-laws!

CLAYTON (SMILING): That's comforting to hear. It certainly seems to me that you're in the midst of a stressful perfect storm.

KEENAN: Whew, that's for sure.

CLAYTON: I realize it's early in the process, but what's been the worst part of all of this for you?

KEENAN: Hmm. With my wife, Melissa, getting laid off in a couple of weeks, and with our company not giving us even a cost-of-living wage increase, right now the worst part seems like the financial uncertainty.

CLAYTON: I can certainly see where that might be the worst part. Any initial thoughts on how you might go about trying to work on or solve this problem?

KEENAN: Well, Melissa hasn't been too happy with where she's been working for a while. In fact, she started looking for other jobs about a month ago, but it's been tough. I don't know how long it might take her to find a job, so I don't know when additional money will be coming in. And with our son being a junior in high school, we're also starting to think and worry about college expenses.

CLAYTON: I'm wondering about that for myself and my family, but my wife isn't being laid off, so I can only imagine how you might be feeling overwhelmed.

KEENAN: That's a good way to put it.

CLAYTON: You know, maybe a better way to put it is that you're feeling out of control.

KEENAN: What makes that a better way to put it?

CLAYTON: Because control is something capable of being managed.

KEENAN: Huh. I wouldn't have thought of it this way.

CLAYTON: You seem to be surrendering your well-being to people and situations outside your control. So, think about the one thing you can control—and that's you.

KEENAN: When did you get so insightful? Is this from doing yoga?

CLAYTON: It has definitely helped me be more aware of myself and stay composed, even under pressure. Here's something else to consider from the person who's credited with developing the concept of stress: It's not what happens to you that matters, it's how you take it.

KEENAN: I'm impressed.

CLAYTON: What have you done in the past to cope with stress? What helps you feel relaxed, safe, and comfortable?

KEENAN: Melissa and I take walks after dinner, and I enjoy woodworking in my basement. I've been there a lot more in the past week with Melissa's parents staying with us, and I can envision myself spending even more time there for at least the next several weeks.

CLAYTON: That sounds like a decent plan. Just wondering—what would you say to me if our situations were reversed?

KEENAN: That seems easy. Given the success you seem to be having with yoga and learning about dealing with stress, I'd say continue with what you're doing for sure. I'm going to start by practicing the breathing.

CLAYTON: Hey, why don't you and Melissa join my wife and me at the yoga class? It's an open, free class sponsored by the community center. We'd love to have you there with us, and you said that the two of you enjoy going for walks after dinner, so the timing sounds right.

KEENAN: Let me talk with her and get back to you tomorrow.

CLAYTON: I'm sorry you're going through this, Keenan, but I'm here to help you. Let's meet again tomorrow to flesh out more of the details. But hopefully this was a reasonably productive start.

KEENAN: It was. I feel better and more hopeful. Thanks, Clayton.

References

American Psychological Association. *Stress in America in 2023: A nation recovering from collective trauma.* https://www.apa.org/news/press/releases/stress/2023/collective-trauma-recovery

Bremner, J. D., Moazzami, K., Wittbrodt, M. T., Nye, J. A., Lima, B. B., Gillespie, C. F., Rapaport, M. H., Pearce, B. D., Shah, A. J., & Vaccarino, V. (2020). Diet, stress and mental health. *Nutrients, 12*(8), 2428. https://doi.org/10.3390/nu12082428

Cannon, W. B. (1939). *The wisdom of the body* (2nd ed.). W. W. Norton.

Choi, S., Nah, S., Jang, H-D., Moon, J. E., & Han, S. (2021). Association between chronic low back pain and degree of stress: A nationwide cross-sectional study. *Scientific Reports, 11,*14549. https://doi.org/10.1038/s41598-021-94001-1

Davidson, L. M., & Baum, A. (1986). Chronic stress and posttraumatic stress disorders. *Journal of Consulting and Clinical Psychology, 54*(3), 303–308. https://doi.org/10/1037/0022-006X.54.3.303

Edwards, M. K., & Loprinzi, P. D. (2017). Comparative effects of meditation and exercise on physical and psychosocial health outcomes: A review of randomized controlled trials. *Postgraduate Medicine, 130*(2), 222–228. https://doi.org/10.1080/00325481.2018.1409049

Everly, G. S., Jr., & Lating, J. M. (2022). *The Johns Hopkins guide to psychological first aid* (2nd ed.). Johns Hopkins University Press.

Freudenberger, H. H. (1984). Impaired clinicians: Coping with burnout. In P. A. Keller & L. Ritt (Eds.), *Innovations in clinical practice: A sourcebook* (Vol. 3, pp. 221–228). Professional Resource Exchange.

Gallup. (2023). *Gallup global emotion 2023: World unhappier, more stressed out than ever.* https://news.gallup.com/poll/394025/world-unhappier -stressed-ever.aspx.

Gao, S., Wang, X., Meng L-b., Zhang, Y-m., Luo, Y., Gong, T., Liu, D-p., Chen, Z-g., & Li, Y-j. (2022). Recent progress of chronic stress in the development of atherosclerosis. *Oxidative Medicine and Cellular Longevity.* https://doi.org/10.1155/2022/4121173

Ghahramani, S., Lankarani, K. B., Yousefi, M., Heydari, K., Shahabi, S., & Azmand, S. (2021). A systematic review and meta-analysis of burnout among healthcare workers during COVID-19. *Frontiers in Psychiatry, 12.* https://do.org/10.3389/fpsyt.2021.758849

Girdano, D. A., Dusek, D. E., & Everly, G. S., Jr. (2013). *Controlling stress and tension* (9th ed.). Pearson.

Hussenoeder, F. X., Conrad, I., Pabst, A., Luppa, M., Stein, J., Engel, C., Zachariae, S., Zeynalova, S., Yahiaoui-Doktor, M., Glaesmer, H., Hinz, A., Witte, V., Wichmann, G., Kirsten, T., Löffler, M., Villringer, A., & Riedel-Hell, S. G. (2022). Different areas of chronic stress and their associations with depression. *Environmental Research and Public Health, 19*(14), 8773. https://doi.org/10.3390/ijerph19148773

Kim, J., Li, L., Korous, K. M., Valiente, C., & Tsethlikai, M. (2022). Chronic stress predicts post-traumatic stress disorder symptoms via executive function deficits among urban American Indian children. *Stress, 25*(1), 97–104. https://doi.org/10.1080/10253890.2021.2024164

Kowal, M., Coll-Martin, T., Ikizer, G., Rasmussen, J., Eichel, K., Studzińska, A., Koszalkowska, K., Karwowski, M., Najmussaqib, A., Pankowski, D., Lieberoth, A., & Ahmed, O. (2020). Who is the most stressed during the COVID-19 pandemic? Data from 26 countries and areas. *Applied Psychology: Health and Well-Being, 12*(4), 946–966. https://doi.org/10.1111/aphw.12234

Labanski, A., Langhorst, J., Engler, H., & Elsenbruch, S. (2020). Stress and the brain-gut axis in functional and chronic-inflammatory gastrointestinal diseases. *Psychoneuroendocrinology, 111,* 104501. https://doi.org/10.1016/j.psyneuen.2019.104501

Liu, M-Y., Li, N., Li, W. A., & Khan, H. (2017). Association between psychosocial stress and hypertension: A systematic review and meta-analysis. *Neurological Research, 39*(6), 573–580. https://doi.org/10.1080/01616412.2017.1317904

Lu, Y., Nyunt, M. S. Z., Gwee, X., Feng, L., Feng, L., Kua, E. H., Kumar, R., & Ng, T. P. (2012). Life event stress and chronic obstructive pulmonary disease (COPD): Associations with mental well-being and quality of life in a population-based study. *BMJ Open, 2,* e001674. https://doi.org/10.1136/bmjopen-2012-001674

McEwen, B. S. (1998). Stress, adaptation, and disease: Allostasis and allostatic load. *Annals of the New York Academy of Sciences, 840*(1), 33–44. https://doi.org/10/1111/j.1749-6632.1998.tb09546.x

McEwen, B. S. (2019). What is the confusion with cortisol? *Chronic Stress, 3.* https://doi.org/10.1177/2470547019833647

McEwen, B. S., & Wingfield, J. C. (2003). The concept of allostasis in biology and biomedicine. *Hormones and Behavior, 43*(1), 2–15. https://doi.org/10.1016/S0018-506X(02)00024-7

Rosenstein, L. S., Edwards, S. T., & Landon, B. E. (2023). Adult primary care physician visits increasingly address mental health concerns. *Health Affairs, 42*(2), 163–171. https//doi.org/10.1377/hlthaff.2022.00705

Salari, N., Khazaie, H., Hosseinian-Far, A., Khaledi-Paveh, K., Kazeminia, M., Mohammadi, M., Sholaima, S., Daneshkhah, A., & Eskandari, S. (2020). The prevalence of stress, anxiety and depression within front-line healthcare workers caring for COVID-19 patients: A systematic review and meta-regression. *Human Resources for Health, 18,* 100. https://doi.org/10/1186/s12960-020-00544-1

Sandberg, S., Paton, J. Y., Ahola, S., McCann, D. C., McGuinness, D., Hillary, C. R., & Oja, H. (2000). The role of acute and chronic stress in asthma attacks in children. *The Lancet, 356,* 982–987. https://doi.org/10.1111/j.1651-2227.2002.tb01687.x.

Schramm, S. H., Moebus, S., Lehmann, N., Galli, U., Obermann, M., Bock, E., Yoon, M-S., Diener, H-C., & Katsarava, Z. (2015). The association between stress and headache. *Cephalagia, 35*(10), 853–863. https://doi.org/10.1177/0333102414563087

Seeman, T. E., McEwen, B. S., Rowe, J. W., & Singer, B. H. (2001). Allostatic load as a marker of cumulative biological risk: MacArthur studies of successful aging. *Proceedings of the National Academy of Sciences, 98*(8), 4770–4775. https://doi.org/10.1073/pnas.081072698

Selye, H. (1956). *The stress of life.* McGraw-Hill.

Sharma, M. (2014). Yoga as an alternative and complementary approach for stress management: A systematic review. *Journal of Evidence-Based Complementary & Alternative Medicine, 19*(1), 59–67. https://doi.org/10.1177/2156587213503344

Sharma, V. K., & Singh, T. G. (2020). Chronic stress and diabetes mellitus: Interwoven pathologies. *Current Diabetes Reviews, 16*(6), 546–556. https://doi.org/10.2174/1573399981566619111152248

World Health Organization. (2019). *Burn-out an "occupational phenomenon": International Classification of Diseases.* https://www.who.int/news/item/28-05-2019-burn-out-an-occupational-phenomenon-international-classification-of-diseases

SEVEN | Fear Of . . .

GRACIELA IS AN INTROVERTED 15-YEAR-OLD *whose family moved into their new home, located 200 miles from their previous one, two weeks ago. There has been a lot of adjusting, and Graciela has not yet met anyone her age in the neighborhood.*

Graciela plans to try out for her new high school's soccer team. She wants to make sure she understands the instructions correctly, so she slowly rereads the email. She writes her last name in four-inch block letters on the back of a white T-shirt, then grabs her bag, her water bottle, and her cleats. Her dad, Ramon, agrees to drive her to the school, which she has never seen.

When they arrive at the parking lot, Graciela asks her dad to park away from the other cars so she can sit for a few minutes. She watches as others, also wearing white T-shirts, eagerly get out of their cars, run to hug each other, and seem genuinely excited to be there.

Graciela, breathing rapidly and with tears in her eyes, turns to her father and says, "Poppy, they'll never accept me. I'm too afraid to get out of the car and do this." What does Ramon say?

What Is Fear?

Fear is the cognitive appraisal of threat coupled with an emotionally aroused, agitated response to a specific real or imagined person, thing, or situation (Gullone, 2000). It might arise when someone is walking over a battered bridge, anticipating a dental procedure, or—as in Graciela's scenario—facing something extremely uncomfortable for the first time and fearing rejection. In most cases, fear activates the body's mobilizing fight-or-flight response (see Chapter Six), though it can also lead to hesitation, or a "freezing" reaction. Fear is a fundamental part of the human condition, helping us respond adaptively to potentially dangerous situations.

In some instances, fear can prevent us from entering a situation that might cause physical or psychological injury. It can also help us decide if, when, and how to leave an encounter that becomes too threatening—or worse. Fear is often an anticipatory emotional state that can linger, creating uneasiness and tension. In most cases, it serves a helpful role by aiding in harm avoidance and "supercharging" one's physical abilities. The fight-or-flight response, for example, temporarily increases strength and speed, and reduces pain sensitivity. That said, fear becomes unhelpful when it keeps you from doing something you really want to do or from taking reasonable risks that might improve your life.

Key Features: Signs and Symptoms

Psychological Symptoms

It is relevant to understand that fear and anxiety (see Chapter Eight) are closely related, and the distinction between the two can be unclear, partly because the terms are often used to define one another (Perusini & Fanselow, 2015). In general, anxiety refers to a lingering, diffuse sense of apprehension and emotional arousal in response to an ambiguous or uncertain situation (Crocq, 2022), whereas fear is considered a more primitive, survival-driven reaction to something specific (such as rejection, failure, spiders, heights, snakes, etc.). The relationship between the two is made even more complex by the fact that when fear becomes disproportionate to the actual threat, it can evolve into maladaptive responses characteristic of anxiety (Perusini et al., 2016). Additionally, extreme fear may escalate into panic (see Chapter Ten). To summarize (and possibly risk oversimplifying): while anxiety tends to involve apprehension and arousal in response to something vague or ambiguous, fear typically involves those reactions in response to something specific.

Physical Symptoms

Once a fear-provoking situation is recognized, it rapidly triggers circuits in the brain's emotional-processing center, known as the limbic system (called a "system" because it consists of multiple interrelated structures). One key element of this system is the amygdala, an almond-shaped structure primarily involved in the learning and expression of fear (Keifer et al., 2015). Once triggered, the amygdala activates another part of the limbic system: the hypothalamus. The hypothalamus then sends signals either directly to target organs for an immediate response, or to the adrenal glands—located on top of the kidneys—which continue the fight-or-flight response by releasing hormones such as adrenaline and cortisol.

The signs and symptoms of a fear response, which are consistent with the fight-or-flight response, include several beneficial effects, such as:

- Rapid heartbeat, which provides more oxygen to muscles
- Increased muscular strength
- Reduced pain sensitivity
- Increased speed
- Increased visual acuity

But fear can also manifest in potentially counterproductive reactions, such as:

- Trembling
- Sweating
- Dry mouth
- Chills
- Nausea
- Confusion
- Dizziness
- Hesitation, freezing in place

From an evolutionary perspective, this rapid biochemical and emotional response, when activated to a moderate degree, enables us to protect ourselves from danger and aids in survival; however, it becomes disabling at higher intensities.

Other brain regions involved in the fear response are the hippocampus, which plays a role in forming memories for factual information, and the prefrontal cortex, the front part of the brain, which is involved in appraisal and decision-making. These two regions collaborate in interpreting fear—helping determine whether our fear response was accurate and justified or if we may have overreacted.

The combination of interpretive, emotional, and biochemical responses helps explain why, in some instances, fear can be associated with other, more enjoyable, emotions. For example, many people seek and enjoy the thrill (i.e., adrenaline rush) of scary movies or roller coasters because their brain has assessed the actual danger and determined it to be limited. But when a situation is appraised as potentially harmful, the intensity of one's reactions increases and may fuel itself, leading to a sense of losing control.

So what's the takeaway? Fear reactions, like stress (see Chapter Six), are often more influenced by how you interpret a situation than by the situation itself. The Greek philosopher Epictetus is credited with noting that we are disturbed not by things, but by the views we take of them. This insight will be useful when we consider how to help people in a fear-based crisis.

Types of Fear

Although terms like "performance anxiety" and "test anxiety" are common in most vocabularies, we have chosen to include them here, alongside the more serious condition of phobias, rather than in the anxiety chapter. Our rationale for this decision is that the specific nature of each condition aligns more closely with the way fear is defined and conceptualized. We briefly touch on panic in the anxiety chapter because it is classified as an anxiety disorder, but given its prevalence, we have also given it a separate chapter (see Chapter Ten).

Performance Anxiety (Fear of Poor Performance)

You're up next! Performance anxiety is fear or worry of being in the spotlight and being unable to successfully complete a task, even if well-prepared. It can occur in any situation where behaviors are socially evaluated, such as acting, singing, dancing, or performing athletically (or sexually), especially when there are real or perceived consequences. Performance anxiety can either enhance functioning (getting "psyched up") or disrupt it (getting "psyched out") (Brooks, 2014). Many individuals with performance anxiety tie their sense of self to their desired skill, and poor performances can lead to concerns about long-term failure (Niering et al., 2023).

Performance anxiety, sometimes referred to as "stage fright" in entertainers, occurs when thinking and memory, including motor memory, are highlighted. In athletes, where visual/spatial and motor responses are emphasized, performance anxiety is often linked to fear of failure, unrealistic expectations (perfectionism, or the inability to execute a task in a way that is acceptable to them), and lack of confidence (Angelidis et al., 2019). Performance anxiety that leads to substandard performance is commonly called "choking under pressure." This can happen from overthinking the task, or "paralysis by analysis." In other cases, fine motor skills can be impacted, resulting in the "yips"—a phenomenon many golfers have experienced.

Several symptoms associated with performance anxiety are listed above. While studies on the prevalence rates of performance anxiety in athletes vary based on the type of activity and levels of experience and expertise, estimates from small, select samples of amateur athletes suggest rates of around 30–60% (Rowland & van Lankveld, 2019). The prevalence of performance anxiety in professional musicians has been reported to range from 16.5% to 60%, with more women than men being affected, and those over 45–50 years old reporting less performance anxiety than younger musicians (Fernholz et al., 2019). In a sample of adolescent musicians, the overall prevalence rate of high performance anxiety was 11% (Papageorgi, 2022).

Performance anxiety is often associated with social anxiety or social phobia (see below). The key difference between the two is that individuals with social anxiety tend to overestimate the extent or significance of being watched or evaluated, whereas performance anxiety usually occurs in the presence of an actual audience that will likely evaluate or judge the quality of a skill that typically requires practice (unlike social interactions, which are a daily activity not generally considered to require practice) (Hofmann et al., 1997; Kenny, 2010). Moreover, those with social anxiety often seek to avoid interactions if they can, whereas individuals with performance anxiety, despite their fear, typically remain committed to the very task that causes them anxiety (Powell, 2004).

Test Anxiety (Test Fear)

It is very common to feel a certain amount of nervousness before taking a test. This discomfort, if not severe before or during the test, may lead to greater focus and attentiveness, potentially improving results. But if the distress becomes extreme, it can impair one's ability to think clearly, resulting in poorer test performance. Test anxiety is a form of performance anxiety that is intrapersonal (how one relates to oneself) instead of interpersonal (relating to others).

There is a snowball effect associated with test anxiety. Once someone begins blanking on answers during a test, it exacerbates the fear and uncertainty, making it even harder to think clearly and access information stored in the prefrontal cortex of the brain. This cycle is particularly frustrating because individuals with test anxiety often know the answers but can't retrieve them in the moment. It is not uncommon, therefore, that after the exam, when the arousal subsides, those with test anxiety are able to recall the answers—but by then it's too late! This not only leads to disappointment about the current performance but also increases fear about the next exam. A study of more than 2,400 adolescent students revealed that 16.4% reported being highly test anxious, with the proportion higher in female students (22.5%) than male students (10.3%) (Putwain & Daly, 2014).

Fear of Failure

Fear of failure, previously noted as a common feature of performance anxiety, is known scientifically as atychiphobia when it becomes excessive. Although not listed in the *DSM-5-TR* (American Psychiatric Association [APA], 2022), it refers to an irrational and persistent fear of making mistakes and failing. It is often related to perfectionism but can also stem from underestimating one's abilities, knowledge, or skills; putting things off (procrastination); self-defeating statements (such as telling yourself or others that you're likely to fail); and concerns about disappointing others. Multiple factors are thought to contribute to fear of failure, including genetics, an upbringing marked by excessive criticism (suggesting a learned behavior), and a history of trauma (Cherry 2023). It's also worth noting — especially in relation to perfectionism and as a recurring theme throughout this manual — that how one interprets failure makes a difference.

Some signs associated with fear of failure include:

- Feeling out of control
- Avoidance
- Indecisiveness
- Irritability
- Pessimism
- Unwillingness to accept constructive criticism

Fear of failure can lead to feelings of depression (see Chapter Five), anxiety (see Chapter Eight), panic attacks (see Chapter Ten), shame (see Chapter Fourteen), and poor self-esteem. In a large study of more than 517,000 15-year-old students from 59 countries, researchers used statements such as "When I am failing, I worry about what others think of me," "When I am failing, I am afraid that I do not have enough talent," "When I am failing, this makes me doubt my plans for the future" to create an index measuring fear of failure. The results showed that female students reported considerably higher levels of fear of failure than male students. High-achieving female students were especially prone to this fear, and being around other high-achieving peers was associated with increased fear of failure among female students, but not among male students (Borgonovi & Han, 2021).

Fear of Rejection

Like other types of fear described in this chapter, most, if not all, people have experienced discomfort and nervousness when put in situations that could lead to rejection. When more extreme, however, this fear can become overwhelming and may contribute to social anxiety, discussed below. Fear of rejection is related to the fear of being judged by others and subsequently excluded.

Fear of rejection is thought to be so common because, from a survival standpoint, humans evolved as social creatures, drawn to communities that offered protection, shelter, and support. Although most of us don't need this level of communal support today, the biological instinct remains. At the same time, humans are wired to avoid pain, including emotional pain. As a result, some people withdraw from situations that might expose them to unpleasant emotions (e.g., dating, applying for a new job, going to parties), avoid asking for help, or refrain from expressing genuine feelings. This withdrawal can be reinforced, if not rationalized, by a tendency to interpret situations and other people negatively. It can be further compounded by how one perceives being excluded or rejected. Those who are especially sensitive are more likely to struggle with low self-worth or self-esteem. In distancing ourselves physically or emotionally from others, we in essence abandon others before they can reject us. Over time, this pattern can lead to social isolation and loneliness.

Likely due to its pervasiveness, there are no clear prevalence data on fear of rejection. However, a recent study of university students found a positive correlation between fear of rejection and problematic social media use, as measured by a social media addiction scale (Klarenbeek, 2023). In a representative sample of more than 5,000 US middle and high school students, about 27% reported having been cyberbullied in the past 30 days. Among those who experienced cyberbullying, 30.4% received mean or hurtful comments online, 28.9% were excluded from group chats, 28.4% had rumors spread about them online, and 26.9% reported that someone had embarrassed or humiliated them online (Cyberbullying Research Center, 2024).

Phobias

When the normal fear response becomes extreme, it can lead to an intense, enduring, and irrational fear or anxiety of a specific object, situation, or event. This is known as a phobia. What triggers fear and the development of phobias, as well as how someone reacts to them, varies considerably. Some researchers have explored possible genetic links to phobias (e.g., a tendency to fear things that posed threats to our ancestors, such as snakes and spiders, or having similar fears as family members) (Fyer et al., 1995; Kendler et al., 1999). Others have examined how phobias are learned through direct experience (e.g., developing a fear of dogs after being bitten) or indirect exposure (e.g., developing a fear of heights because your father has a fear of heights) (Singh, & Singh, 2016). People with phobias are often highly distressed by the prospect of encountering the feared situation or object and may go to great lengths to avoid it.

As noted previously, although phobias are classified as anxiety disorders in *DSM-5-TR* (APA, 2022), we included them in this chapter due to their specific nature. There are various types of phobias; some of the most common are listed below:

- *Specific phobias* involve an unrealistic or extreme fear of a specific situation, object, or setting, such as a fear of snakes, spiders, heights, airplanes, or blood. In the United States, rates of specific phobias are as high as 12.5% (Kessler et al., 2005). A survey of 22 countries involving nearly 125,000 respondents found that 7.4% reported experiencing specific phobias at some point in their lifetime, and 5.5% experienced a specific phobia within the past 12 months, with females reporting higher rates than males (Wardenaar et al., 2017). Fear of heights is the most common specific phobia, while the fear of being alone is considered the most debilitating for those who experience it (Depla et al., 2008).
- *Social phobia* is a fear of being scrutinized, judged harshly, or humiliated in public situations. The term "social phobia" has been updated to "social anxiety" in the *DSM-5-TR*, so its prevalence is discussed in the anxiety chapter (Chapter Eight).
- *Agoraphobia* is a disproportionate fear of certain environments, most commonly public spaces. The worldwide lifetime prevalence of agoraphobia is around 1.5%, based on a survey of over 136,000 participants from 27 countries (Roest et al., 2019), which is consistent with the prevalence rate of 1.3% in the United States (Harvard Medical School, 2007).

Phobias with Panic

Phobia fear reactions are sometimes accompanied by panic. While panic is addressed in the anxiety chapter (see Chapter Eight) and covered in its own chapter (see Chapter Ten), mentioning it here seems appropriate. Panic refers to an acute, seemingly uncontrollable sense of fear or anxiety typically fueled by irrational thoughts. People experiencing panic commonly feel out of control and as if they are suffocating. The psychology of panic is accompanied by activation of the body's sympathetic nervous system, leading to the fight-or-flight response, which results in elevated heart rate, blood pressure, and muscle tension. In some cases, the parasympathetic nervous system is triggered, causing a dramatic decline in blood pressure that can result in syncope (fainting).

Panic Versus Choking Under Pressure

The terms "choke" and "panic" are often used to describe performance reactions in high-pressure situations. Although the processes that create them are vastly different, they both arise from a fear of failure. And their respective remedies are very different.

"Choking under pressure" refers to a situation where someone fails to perform to their usual standard due to the pressure of the moment. It occurs when a person has the necessary skills and capability, but their performance deteriorates under stress. For example, an athlete missing an easy shot during an important match due to overthinking or fear of failure is said to choke. Notable examples include Greg Norman's performance at the 1996 Masters golf tournament, where he lost a six-shot lead on the final round, or Jana Novotná's performance in the 1993 Wimbledon tennis final against Steffi Graf, where Novotná lost in the final set after leading 4–1 and winning the second set 6–1. The remedy for choking under pressure is to return to overlearned behaviors—those that do not require analysis but rather come naturally after study, rehearsal, and practice.

Panic, on the other hand, in this context, is a more intense and overwhelming response to accumulating stress. It is characterized by a loss of control, where a person may act irrationally or fail to act at all. Panic often involves a sudden onset of fear or anxiety that disrupts normal functioning. Unlike choking, which is a decline in performance, panic is about losing the ability to think or act clearly in the face of stress. The remedy for panic under pressure is to slow down, take a few deep breaths, and think through the situation and the required response, remembering that while you can't always control the situation, you can control how you react to it.

In summary, choking is about performing below one's usual level due to pressure, while panic is about losing control or reacting irrationally due to intense fear or anxiety. Author Malcom Gladwell (2000) insightfully illuminated the difference between the two in his article "The Art of Failure": "Choking is about thinking too much. Panic is about thinking too little. Choking is about loss of instinct. Panic is reversion to instinct."

Potential E-PFA Recommendations
(Think About Trying This)

What should Ramon say to Graciela? What would you say if you were in Ramon's position or one similar?

The five-step E-PFA intervention remains fundamentally the same as we have seen in other chapters:

1) Introduce yourself (if applicable), offer to help, set expectations, de-escalate (if needed).
2) Gather information. (*What happened? What hurts? How bad is it?*)
3) Clarify. (*What's the worst part?*)
4) Provide assistance. (*What do you need right now? How can I help?*)
    a. *Can Ramon use problem-focused assistance?*
    b. *Can Ramon use emotion-focused assistance?*
    c. *Can Ramon use stress management?*
5) Make a plan. (*Next steps?*)

Introduce Yourself, Offer to Help, Set Expectations, De-escalate

- The first step for Ramon might be to help lower the stress Graciela is experiencing in the moment. This is the time for him to be a calm and reassuring presence.

Gather Information

- Graciela is resisting getting out of the car. (*What happened?*) She has expressed feeling "afraid," and it is clear that she fears rejection. She is worried the other girls will not accept her. (*What hurts?*) Her fear has left her frozen, unwilling to go to the tryouts. Ramon may recognize that if this continues, her resistance could keep her from joining the team. (*How bad?*)

Clarify

- Ramon can paraphrase and clarify that Graciela's fear is about being accepted—not about her soccer skills—which is likely an important distinction.
- He can acknowledge that we all want to be accepted, and we all at one time or another have feared rejection.

Provide Assistance

- Ramon can ask Graciela, "What do you need right now?" or "How can I help?" If going further seems warranted, he can offer more direct assistance, as described next. If Ramon is unsure where to begin, Graciela's response to the question about "the worst part" might help him decide.

Problem-Focused

- In task-oriented groups, social acceptance is often based not only on social skills but also on performance relevant to the task. In this case, Graciela's soccer skills are far more likely to earn acceptance than her social adeptness. Can she "earn" the other girls' acceptance through how well she plays? Here, Ramon can help shift her focus from something she cannot control (other girls' opinions) to something she can (her effort and performance on the field). This approach assumes Graciela feels confident in her soccer skills. If that's not the case, Ramon might instead take a more emotion-focused approach.

Emotion-Focused

- Ramon can explain to Graciela that the stress she feels is her body's way of getting supercharged. He can encourage her to channel that emotional energy into her game—using it to play with more focus, intensity, or determination.

Stress Management–Focused

- Ramon can encourage Graciela to "control what she can and cope with the rest." Fear of failure assumes that failure is unacceptable. A powerful cognitive reinterpretation that can be useful in managing this stress is to adopt a mindset that may seem counterintuitive: "Anything worth having is worth failing for." By embracing this empowering perspective, Graciela can shift her focus from the outcome to the process. In this light, the only way to fail is to not try.

Make a Plan

- Before Graciela gets out of the car, Ramon can ask what she plans to say to herself to help harness her newfound energy.

E-PFA Dialogue (It Might Sound Like This)

RAMON (CALMLY): I understand you're afraid, Graciela. To be honest, I'd be more surprised if you weren't.

GRACIELA: Really.

RAMON: Yeah, I'm nervous for you too. In a new situation like this, it's to be expected. Do you feel kinda stuck or frozen?

GRACIELA: Yeah, pretty much.

RAMON: Let's take a couple of deep breaths and focus on something else to help you get unstuck. Breath in through your nose and slowly out through your mouth. And while you're breathing, close your eyes and see yourself out on the field . . . right over there, collecting the ball, keeping your head up, and looking for a good pass to make. Let me know when you can see it.

GRACIELA (WITH HER EYES CLOSED AND AFTER SLOWLY EXHALING): I'm starting to see it.

RAMON: Good. If it helps, think of all the times we practiced together and how well you played on your last team. I'm thinking of that breakaway goal you had that helped your team in the final game of the regional tournament. You played so well that day. Think about and focus on how you can play like that today.

GRACIELA (STOPPING THE DEEP BREATHING AND OPENING HER EYES): I'm okay with my ability to play.

RAMON: Ah, I see. You also mentioned that you're afraid they might not accept you. Is that part of your concern?

GRACIELA: A big part.

RAMON: So, your fear is not about your soccer skills; it's more about being accepted?

GRACIELA: Yeah.

RAMON: We all want to be accepted, Graciela. And everyone at one time or another has feared rejection, including me.

GRACIELA: You?

RAMON: Of course. When I started my new job two weeks ago, I wanted to be liked and accepted. It's part of being human. But you know, feeling confident about my ability to do the job helps with acceptance. And it seems to me, the same strategy can work for you.

GRACIELA: Huh. What do you mean?

RAMON: You're confident in your soccer skills, so let them do the initial "talking." You can earn acceptance from making a good pass, talking on the field, and encouraging others—you know, being a good teammate.

GRACIELA: But what if these girls are really, really good? Who knows—they could have all played on the same club team.

RAMON: That's certainly a possibility, but every team wants as many good players—and just as importantly, as many good teammates—as it can get.

GRACIELA: Hmm. I hear you. And I'm feeling less frozen. But I have a lot of nervous energy.

RAMON: Of course you do. The stressful energy you're describing is helping to get your body supercharged. You can harness that emotional energy to help you play even better.

GRACIELA (TAKING A QUICK, DEEP BREATH AND FORCEFULLY EXHALING): I hope so.

RAMON: Remember, Graciela, control what you can and cope with the rest. I know what happens on the field might not be as relevant as the effort you're about to make to get out of this car to find out. The only real way to fail in this instance is not to try.

GRACIELA: Thanks, Poppy. I'm gonna do this.

RAMON: What are you going to say to yourself to help you harness your newfound energy?

GRACIELA (PAUSING): I'm already so fortunate to be a part of a great family team that loves and accepts me. I'm ready to work on becoming a part of this new team.

RAMON (WORKING TO CONCEAL HIS EMOTIONS): Go have fun.

References

American Psychiatric Association. (2022). Anxiety disorders. In *Diagnostic and statistical manual of mental disorders* (5th ed., text rev.). https://doi.org/10.1176/appi.books.9780890425787.x05_Anxiety _Disorders

Angelidis, A., Solis, E., Lautenbach, F., van der Does, W., & Putman, P. (2019). I'm going to fail! Acute cognitive performance anxiety increases threat-interference and impairs WM performance. *PLOS One, 14*(2). https://doi.org/10.1371/journal.pone.0210824

Borgonovi, F., & Han, S. W. (2021). Gender disparities in fear of failure among 15-year-old students: The role of gender inequality, the organisation of schooling economic conditions. *Journal of Adolescence, 86*, 28–39. https://doi.org/10.1016/j.adolescence.2020.11.009

Brooks, A. W. (2014). Get excited: Reappraising pre-performance anxiety as excitement. *Journal of Experimental Psychology: General, 143*(3), 1144–1158. https://doi.org/10.1037/a0035325

Cherry, K. (2023). *How to deal with the fear of failure.* Verywellmind. https://www.verywellmind.com/what-is-the-fear-of-failure -5176202

Crocq, M.-A. (2022). The history of generalized anxiety as a diagnostic category. *Dialogues in Clinical Neuroscience, 19*(2), 107–115. https://doi.org/10.31887/DCNS.2017.19.2/macrocq

Cyberbullying Research Center. (2024). *2023 Cyberbullying data.* https://cyberbullying.org/2023-cyberbullying-data

Depla, M. F. I. A., ten Have, M. I., van Balkom, A. J. L. M., & de Graaf, R. (2008). Specific fears and phobias in the general population: Results from the Netherlands Mental Health Survey and Incidence Study (NEMESIS). *Social Psychiatry and Psychiatric Epidemiology, 43,* 200–208. https://doi.org/10.1007/s00127-007-0291-z

Fernholz, I., Mumm, J. L. M., Plag, J., Noeres, K., Rotter, G., Willich, S. N., Ströhle, A., Berghöfer, A., & Schmidt, A. (2019). Performance anxiety in professional musicians: A systematic review on prevalence, risk factors and clinical treatment effects. *Psychological Medicine, 49*(14), 2287–2306. https://doi.org/10.1017/S003329 1719001910

Fyer, A. J., Mannuzza, S., & Chapman, T. F. (1995). Specificity in familial aggregation of phobic disorders. *Archives of General Psychiatry, 52,* 564–573. https://doi.org/10.1001/archpsyc.1995.03950190046007

Gladwell, M. (2000, August 21 & 28). The art of failure. *New Yorker.*

Harvard Medical School. (2007). *National Comorbidity Survey (NCS).* https://www.hcp.med.harvard.edu/ncs/index.php

Hofmann, S. G., Gerlach, A. L., Wender, A., & Roth, W. T. (1997). Speech disturbances and gaze behavior during public speaking in subtypes of social phobia. *Journal of Anxiety Disorders, 11*(6), 573–585. https://doi.org?10.1016/S0887-6185

Keifer, O., Jr., Hurt, R. C., Ressler, & K. J., Marvar, P. J. (2015). The physiology of fear: Reconceptualizing the role of the central amygdala in fear learning. *Physiology, 30*(5), 389–401. https://doi.org/10.1152/physiol.00058.2014

Kendler, K. S., Karkowski, L. M., & Prescott, C. A. (1999). Fears and phobias: Reliability and heritability. *Psychological Medicine, 29*(3), 539–553. https://doi.org/10.1017/S0033291799008429

Kenny, D. T. (2010). The role of negative emotions in performance anxiety. In P. Juslin & J. Sloboda (Eds.), *Handbook of music and emotion: Theory, research, applications* (pp. 425–452). Oxford University Press.

Kessler, R. C., Berglund, P., Demler, O., Jin, R., Merikangas, K. R., & Walters, E. E. (2005). Lifetime prevalence and age-of-onset distributions of DSM-IV disorders in the national comorbidity survey replication. *Archives of General Psychiatry, 62*(6), 593–602. https://doi.org/10.1001/archpsyc.62.6.593

Klarenbeek, M. J. (2023). *The relationships between fear of rejection, perceived social support and problematic social media use.* University of Twente Student Theses. https://essay.utwente.nl/95350/

Niering, M., Monsberger, T., Seifert, J., & Muehlauer T. (2023). Effects of psychological interventions on performance anxiety in performing artists and athletes: A systematic review with meta-analysis. *Behavioral Sciences, 13*(11), 910. https://doi.org/10.3390/bs13110910

Papageorgi, I. (2022). Prevalence and predictors of music performance anxiety in adolescent learners: Contributions of individual, task-related and environmental factors. *Musicae Scientiae, 26*(1), 101–122. https://doi.org/10.1177/1029864920923128

Perusini, J. N., & Fanselow, M. S. (2015). Neurobehavioral perspectives on the distinction between fear and anxiety. *Learning & Memory, 22,* 417–425. https://doi.org/10.1101/lm.039180.115

Perusini, J. N., Meyer, E. M., Long, V. A., Rau, V., Nocera, N., Avershal, J., Maksymetz, J., Spigelman, I., & Fanselow, M. S. (2016). Induction and expression of fear sensitization caused by acute traumatic stress. *Neuropsychopharmacology, 41,* 45–57. https://doi.org/10.1038/npp.2015.224

Powell, D. H. (2004). Treating individuals with debilitating performance anxiety: An introduction. *Journal of Clinical Psychology, 60*(8), 801–808. https://doi.org/10.1002/jclp.20038

Putwain, D., & Daly, A. L. (2014). Test anxiety prevalence and gender differences in a sample of English secondary school students. *Educational Studies, 40*(5), 554–570. https://doi.org/10.1080/03055698.2014.953914

Roest, A. M., de Vries, Y. A., Lim, C. C. W., Wittchen, H.-U., Stein, D. J., Adamowski, T., Al-Hamzawi, A., Bromet, E. J., Viana, M. C., de Girolamo, G., Demyttenaere, K., Florescu, S., Gureje, O., Haro, J. M., Hu, C., Karam, E. G., Caldas-de-Almeida, J. M., Kawakami, N., Lépine, J. P., . . . de Jonge, P. (2019). A comparison of *DSM-5* and *DSM-IV* agoraphobia in the World Health Surveys. *Depression and Anxiety, 36,* 499–510. https://doi.org/10.1002/da.22885

Rowland, D. L., & van Lankveld, J. J. D. M. (2019). Anxiety and performance in sex, sport, and stage: Identifying common ground. *Frontiers in Psychology, 10,* 1615. https://doi.org/10.3389/fpsyg.2019.01615

Singh, J., & Singh, J. (2016). Treatment options for specific phobias. *International Journal of Basic and Clinical Pharmacology, 5*(3), 593–598. https://doi.org/10.18203/2319-2003.ijbcp20161496

Wardenaar, K. J., Lim, C. C. W., Al-Hamzawi, A. O., Alonso, J., Andrade, L. H., Benjet, C., Bunting, B., de Girolamo, G., Demyttenaere, K., Florescu, S. E., Gureje, O., Hisateru, T., Hu, C., Huang, Y., Karam, E., Kiejna, A., Lepine, J. P., Navarro-Mateu, F., Oakley Browne, M., . . . de Jonge, P. (2017). The cross-national epidemiology of specific phobia in the World Mental Health Surveys. *Psychological Medicine, 47*(10), 1744–1760. https://doi.org/10.1017/S0033291717000174

EIGHT | Anxiety

IT'S AFTER 11:30 P.M. ON A FRIDAY, *and 48-year-old Tasha is trying to turn it off. She gets out of bed, walks downstairs, opens and closes the refrigerator door, then walks back upstairs. As she climbs back in bed, she still can't turn it off.*

What is "it"? Apprehension and worry. Tasha is having difficulty falling asleep because her mind is so active. Her legs feel like they're cramping, and she feels increasingly nauseous. Tasha often feels this way—her mind jumping from one topic to another—but tonight she keeps returning to think about relationships. She and her husband divorced two years ago, and earlier today her friend Kaila encouraged her to consider dating again. Now Tasha is thinking, and worrying, about whether she should. Tasha would like to be in a relationship someday, but the uncertainty makes her anxious.

Kaila said she would come to Tasha's apartment the next morning to help with her dating profile. But Tasha is worried that she is not good with computers, won't be able to use the website, and won't know what to write in her profile. She frets that she doesn't have any good photos of herself because she's not photogenic. She starts imagining what it might be like to be on a date and have to make conversation with someone who might think she's unintelligent, unengaging, or unattractive. She begins to feel overwhelmed about both the financial and the emotional demands of dating.

After several hours of restlessness and worry—about dating and many other random topics—Tasha finally gets to sleep. She wakes up feeling a bit groggy. When Kaila arrives, Tasha opens the door looking shaken and agitated. Before Kaila can sit down, Tasha says, "There's no way I'm going to be able to do online dating. It's too complicated, it's too unknown, I'm not going to be successful, and I'm never going to find anyone. What were we thinking?" How does Kaila respond?

What Is Anxiety?

Anxiety is an emotional state marked by extensive feelings of worry, doubt, conflict, and uneasiness (Vanin, 2008). Simply put, it is a state of uncertainty. Most, if not all, of us occasionally worry about things like family issues, health, impending deadlines, and finances. In this way, anxiety is a part of life. And when it's not excessive, anxiety can be motivating. For example, some degree of anxiety has been associated with persistence, academic achievement, and job satisfaction (Strack et al., 2017). Anxiety, then, is complex. It serves different functions, is expressed in different ways, and has a lot of individual variability. The goal of dealing with anxiety, therefore, is to manage it.

Anxiety is different from fear, although the two share similarities (see Chapter Seven). Fear involves arousal and apprehension in response to a specific threat or stressor. This focused response is functionally adaptive: It helps us recognize and respond to real dangers and can help us manage our lives. Anxiety, by contrast, is typically marked by arousal and emotion not tied to a specific threat. Instead, it is more diffuse, free-floating, and anticipatory, again reflecting that core sense of uncertainty (Barlow, 2002). The ambiguous and potentially pervasive nature of anxiety makes it challenging to manage. When it becomes overwhelming, it can interfere with daily life and become debilitating (National Institute of Mental Health, n.d.).

Tasha's current anxiety is surfacing as concern about dating, but it's the more diffuse dread of uncertainty that is the real issue. Next time, she will show her underlying anxiety as worrying about something else. And this pattern will likely repeat itself. As you read the rest of the chapter, keep in mind that the E-PFA model is equally applicable to less clearly recognized anxiety-producing situations.

Key Features: Signs and Symptoms

While these lists are not comprehensive, here are some key features that can help you recognize anxiety (American Psychiatric Association [APA], 2022).

Cognitive (Thinking) Symptoms

- Difficulty concentrating
- Hyperalertness to overestimated potential future threats
- Repeated, obsessive thoughts (i.e., overthinking past events or anticipating future problems)
- Worry that becomes difficult to control and interferes with daily functioning (e.g., work, social relationships, decision-making)

Physical Symptoms

- Recurrent muscle tension, which can lead to tightness or discomfort
- Fatigue

- Elevated heart rate
- Sweating
- Gastrointestinal problems
- Chronic aches and pains, including headaches

Behavioral Symptoms

- Sleep disturbance (including getting to sleep)
- Avoiding places and situations to prevent uncomfortable feelings
- Restlessness, an inability to relax
- Being on edge, irritability

Prevalence of Anxiety

According to the World Health Organization (2023), anxiety disorders affected more than 301 million people worldwide in 2019, making them the most prevalent emotional disorder globally. In the United States, the US Department of Health and Human Services (Terlizzi & Villarroel, 2020) reported that more than 15% of US adults experienced mild, moderate, or severe anxiety when assessed over a two-week period in 2019. During the COVID-19 pandemic, an estimated 76.2 million additional cases of anxiety disorders were reported worldwide, a 25.6% increase over pre-COVID levels (Santomauro et al., 2021). Also of note, a global study of more than 275,000 adolescents (ages 12–17) found that factors such as being identified as female, being older, having a lower socioeconomic status, and lacking close friends were associated with a greater risk of anxiety and suicidal ideation (see Chapter Sixteen) (Biswas et al., 2020).

Types of Anxiety

The *DSM-5-TR* defines many different anxiety disorders (APA, 2022). While some, such as phobias and panic attacks, are covered in other chapters, here is a brief overview of a few other types of anxiety that may also require a PFA response.

Generalized Anxiety

Generalized anxiety (GA) is a persistent, excessive worry that occurs more days than not for at least six months and covers a range of concerns (e.g., work, school, relationships). Individuals with GA often describe feeling that they have limited control over their free-floating worry, which leads to significant distress or impairment in functioning. This is what we commonly think of when considering someone who is chronically anxious. In a study of around 150,000 adults from 26 countries, the lifetime prevalence of generalized anxiety disorder (GAD) was found to be 3.7% (Ruscio et al., 2017). In the United States, the lifetime risk of GAD is around 9%, with women and girls being more than twice as likely as men and boys to experience it (Kessler et al., 2012; Ruscio et al., 2017).

Separation Anxiety

Separation anxiety involves excessive fear and distress when separated from important people (i.e., attachment figures) in one's life. This includes distress about being away from home or attachment figures, concern that something will happen to the attachment figure (such as injury, illness, or death) while apart, or concern that something similar will happen to oneself if not with the attachment figure. It can also lead to reluctance to leave the house and go to school or work. Although separation anxiety occurs in about 4% of children and around 7.6% of clinical samples

(Battaglia, 2015), it also affects adults, with a lifetime prevalence of up to 6.6% (Bögels et al., 2013).

Panic

A panic attack is defined by the *DSM-5-TR* as "an abrupt surge of intense fear or discomfort" that reaches a peak within minutes (APA, 2022). It involves a sudden and intense (i.e., paroxysmal) discharge of the sympathetic (fight-or-flight) nervous system. In a nationally representative National Comorbidity study, 2.7% of adults aged 15–54 years had experienced panic disorder in the past year, and 4.7% had experienced it at some point in their lives. The prevalence was higher among females (3.8%) than males (1.6%) (Harvard Medical School, 2007). Signs and symptoms of panic include:

- Palpitations, pounding heart, or accelerated heart rate
- Sweating
- Trembling or shaking
- Shortness of breath or feeling of smothering
- Feelings of choking
- Chest pain or discomfort
- Nausea or abdominal distress
- Feeling dizzy, unsteady, light-headed, or faint
- Chills or heat sensations
- Paresthesia (numbness or tingling sensations)

We will cover panic separately in Chapter Ten.

Selective Mutism

Selective mutism is a consistent inability or reluctance to speak in social situations, such as at school, with either children or adults, despite having the language skills and ability to speak. It is often associated with excessive shyness and fear of embarrassment. The prevalence is thought to be low, less than 2% (Muris & Ollendick, 2015), but is noted to be slightly higher in immigrant populations (Elizur & Perednik, 2003).

Potential E-PFA Recommendations
(Think About Trying This)

What should Kaila do to help Tasha? What would you do if you were challenged to help someone in a situation similar to Tasha's? Let's consider her situation through the five-phase E-PFA lens. Listed below are potential E-PFA interventions that Kaila might enlist, depending on the specific details of Tasha's situation.

1) Introduce yourself (if applicable), offer to help, set expectations, de-escalate (if needed).
2) Gather information. (*What happened? What hurts? How bad is it?*)
3) Clarify. (*What's the worst part?*)
4) Provide assistance. (*What do you need right now? How can I help?*)
   a. *Can Kaila use problem-focused assistance?*
   b. *Can Kaila use emotion-focused assistance?*
   c. *Can Kaila use stress management?*
5) Make a plan. (*Next steps?*)

Introduce Yourself, Offer to Help, Set Expectations, De-escalate

- PFA begins with Kaila showing up emotionally, expressing concern, and letting Tasha know that she wants to help. And if Kaila can't help, she will assist Tasha in finding the help she needs. (There is no need for an introduction because the two are already acquainted.)
- In this example, physically visiting with Tasha is the preferred method of contact. Showing up to assist reduces the sense of isolation and shows that somebody cares. But if physically contact-

ing Tasha were not possible, Zoom or FaceTime can be effective. A telephone call would be a last resort but could still be effective.

- Kaila is walking into a highly charged situation in which Tasha appears agitated. Although it is not always needed, an attempt at de-escalation by Kaila may be very useful in this case. Before responding to Tasha's last question — "What were we thinking?" — Kaila could simply say in a calm and reassuring manner, "Okay, let's slow down. How about if we sit down and take a deep breath? Then you can tell me what's going on."

- Psychological "grounding" techniques are also useful in reducing the acute stress associated with anxiety and fear, especially in mitigating panic. Grounding is a form of distraction that Kaila could use to encourage Tasha to focus on something other than her anxious thoughts. This might involve sensory grounding, such as having Tasha focus on a spot on the wall or feel her feet on the floor. Or Kaila could ask Tasha to count backward from 100 by threes or have her count her breaths.

Gather Information

- Having attempted to de-escalate the situation, Kaila could encourage verbal venting or catharsis. Questions like, "So, what's happened? What's going on?" would allow Tasha to talk about the anxiety she is experiencing. (*What happened?*)

- Once Tasha describes the details of her anxious episode, Kaila could ask how her anxiety is affecting her or how it is making her feel. (*What hurts?*)

- Unless it is already clear, Kaila should then inquire about the overall severity of Tasha's anxiety. For example, "This sounds really distressing. How bad is it? How is this disrupting your life?" Remember, severity is defined by the interaction of intensity, urgency, and duration. (*How bad is it?*)

Clarify

- The clarification phase will likely begin with Kaila paraphrasing or recapping what she's heard. For example, "Dating at our age can be really scary. And it sounds like you're not feeling too confident about the whole process." Then she could ask, "So, what's the worst part of this for you?" Or, "How much is this bothering you?" Kaila should listen carefully to Tasha's answer as it will provide some idea about where to start offering further support beyond the active listening she's already done. (*What's the worst part?*)

Provide Assistance

- Kaila can ask Tasha what she needs most right now. She could also ask how Tasha has managed stress in the past, or simply ask how she can help. If this nondirective approach fails to help, Kaila might adopt a more directive approach, using one or more of the suggested focused strategies below. If unsure where to begin, Kaila can use Tasha's response to the question regarding "the worst part" as her starting point.

Problem-Focused

- It would be natural for Tasha to want to run away from the challenges of dating. While not submitting a profile to the dating website would reduce her immediate anxiety, it wouldn't help with her long-term goal of finding a new relationship. Therefore, Kaila should discourage Tasha from avoiding dating altogether.
- Kaila could discuss with Tasha the option of slowing down the dating process. For example, they could divide the process into smaller, more manageable steps. Writing a profile, selecting pictures, and choosing the best dating sites can each be approached slowly and thoughtfully, one at a time.

Emotion-Focused

- Tasha's anxiety is getting in the way of her finding a new relationship. It is a barrier. Perhaps Kaila could help her see how pessimistic she sounds before even beginning the process, and how that pessimism will make things harder than they need to be.
- Tasha might believe she is the only person to feel this way. Kaila can encourage her to talk to other friends and family members, perhaps seeking helpful suggestions on handling self-doubt.
- Kaila can help Tasha redefine success. Sometimes dating, meeting new people, or going to new places can be goals in and of themselves. Seen in this light, there is no such thing as failure.
- Kaila can ask Tasha what she is saying to herself about the situation, reflecting back on what the "worst part" might be.
- Kaila can ask Tasha what she might say to Kaila if their situations were reversed (role reversal).

Stress Management-Focused

- Kaila can remind Tasha that exercise has been shown to improve mood and self-confidence and reduce anxiety.
- She can encourage Tasha to get out of her apartment. Fatigue and loneliness can fuel anxiety.
- Kaila can let Tasha know that early mornings and late nights are likely to be the most difficult times of day for her.

Make a Plan

If something doesn't get scheduled, it doesn't get done. Because Tasha is Kaila's friend, some form of follow-up seems reasonable.

- Kaila can help Tasha develop an antianxiety plan, perhaps addressing issues of uncertainty or fears of rejection.
- Kaila should discuss with Tasha the possibility of getting some professional assistance. There are websites and even online coaches who might be able to help Tasha.

- Kaila can ask Tasha to discuss her anxiety with her primary care physician if it persists or worsens.
- Kaila should check in with Tasha in the next couple of days or so to see how she is doing and if she has sought further support.

E-PFA Dialogue (It Might Sound Like This)

KAILA: There's a lot going on Tasha. Is it okay if we slow down?

TASHA: I'm sorry. I'm overwhelmed with all this, and I didn't sleep well last night.

KAILA: How about we sit down and take a few deep breaths? Then you can tell me what's going on.

TASHA: Yeah, that's a good idea (both taking a seat).

KAILA (AFTER A PAUSE): Take a moment, Tasha, and focus on your breathing . . . in through your nose and out through your mouth. In fact, it might be helpful if you count your breaths.

TASHA (BREATHING AND COUNTING FOR FIVE BREATHS): Ahh . . . I needed that!

KAILA: So, what's happened? What's going on since we last spoke?

TASHA: After we decided to meet this morning and work on my dating profile, I started to think more and more about it and began spinning out of control.

KAILA: Spinning out of control? Tell me more.

TASHA: I'm too old to start dating again. I'm not that interesting, and I don't want to be humiliated. Besides, I don't know what to say in my profile, and the last good picture of me was taken 10 years ago. What if my boss finds out that I'm on a dating sight?

KAILA: Wow, that's a lot. I appreciate you sharing all this, Tasha. How has this been affecting you?

TASHA: I had a terrible time getting to sleep last night, and my mind kept racing to all sorts of different things, including my job and finances. My legs started cramping, and I felt like I was going to get sick.

KAILA: I'm sorry, Tasha. This all sounds distressing.

TASHA: It is.

KAILA: How bad is it?

TASHA: I don't think I want to go through with dating.

KAILA: Let's face it, dating at any age can be challenging, but dating at our age can be downright scary. It sounds like you're not feeling too confident about the whole process, including how your boss might react.

TASHA: I realize that my boss will be supportive. I said that because it all just seems so overwhelming!

KAILA: I genuinely hear what you're saying. I do. What's the worst part?

TASHA: Honestly, like the unknown, I don't have confidence in myself, and I think it's better if I just leave dating alone.

KAILA: What do you need right now? How can I help?

TASHA: Thanks, but I'm not sure.

KAILA: I appreciate you sharing that you don't feel confident. Uncertainty can make us feel uncomfortable and like we want to run away. I get that not submitting a dating profile might feel like a way to ease your anxiety right now, but it's not going to get you any closer to your long-term goal of finding a new relationship. And you deserve that! So I really don't think you should avoid dating altogether.

TASHA: I hear what you're saying, but, like most things in my life, the process seems so huge and unknown.

KAILA: If you consider the process in its entirety, I agree that it might seem huge and unknown. But how about if we slow the process down?

TASHA: What do you mean?

KAILA: Let's divide it into smaller steps. Let's start by finding a few good dating sites, then write a profile, and then make sure we have good pictures to capture your outer beauty. We can do this slowly, one step at a time.

TASHA: I hear you, and I like the idea. But I've been away from dating for too long, and I'm worried that I'm not what people are looking for. I'm really not that interesting, and I doubt if I will get much attention.

KAILA: Tasha, I realize the leap back into dating is challenging, but what I'm hearing right now sounds like your anxiety doing the talking. And the self-doubt is currently getting in the way of what you say you want, which is finding a new relationship. We haven't even looked at dating sites yet, and you're already sounding pessimistic about the outcome. Being unsure and hesitant will make this challenging process even more daunting and harder than it needs to be.

TASHA: I don't get how others are able to do this.

KAILA: That's a valid statement, but one you can assess.

TASHA: What do you mean?

KAILA: Do you know how many people nowadays use dating
sites to meet someone else? I've heard that it's the main way
for people to meet each other. So you're not alone in this;
that's for sure. Why don't you talk to other friends, coworkers,
and your family. I'll bet you know a lot of people who have
used dating sites; you just haven't thought of it.

TASHA (AFTER A 20-SECOND PAUSE): You know . . . as a
matter of fact, I believe my boss met her current partner on a
dating sight.

KAILA: There ya go. It's out there for sure. You could also ask
others for tips and suggestions about handling your self-
doubt, particularly related to dating. In a more general sense,
there are probably some really good self-help books on the
topic of returning to dating.

TASHA: Maybe you're right. I'm letting my worries and uncertainty interfere with what I'm really interested in, and that's
finding a relationship.

KAILA: Good for you to recognize this.

TASHA: But what if I'm not successful?

KAILA: Hmmm . . . you know, it might be helpful to rethink
what success in dating means for you. You love going to new
restaurants and traveling. You also enjoy meeting—not
necessarily dating—people. So maybe these should be your
initial goals—visiting new restaurants and learning about
people you don't know. And Tasha, if you agree with these as
goals, then there is no failure. If you meet some interesting
people along the way, that's a plus. And if you find someone
you really like, that's quite the bonus.

TASHA: I like that reinterpretation. It makes sense and is worth
considering.

KAILA: Tasha, if the roles were reversed and I was in your situation, what would you say to me?

TASHA (CHUCKLING): Oh, I'd most likely be saying the same thing—you know that. But it's always easier when it's someone else going through something. But you're in a great relationship, so I guess it's my turn now. I just need to work on not letting my uncertainty and self-doubt . . . ugh, my anxiety . . . get the better of me.

KAILA: There are other ways to deal with uncertainty and feelings of anxiety. Remember that exercise is a great way to improve mood and burn off some of the excess chemicals that our bodies release when we're anxious.

TASHA: Thanks for the reminder, Kaila. I'm going to go spin class later at the gym. Let me know if you'd like to join me.

KAILA: That sounds good. Also, it's just good to get out of your apartment. Being by yourself, particularly if you're feeling lonely and fatigued, can make anxiety worse. And be aware that early mornings, like now, and late in the evening, when you're trying to sleep, can often be the most challenging.

TASHA: You're right, Kaila. Thanks for taking the time and providing so much insight.

KAILA: Before we finish, let's make sure we have a plan. We both know that if it doesn't get scheduled, it doesn't get done.

TASHA: That's a good idea. And you know I like to be organized . . . maybe at times a bit too much.

KAILA: If you're ready, let's start by looking at dating sites and then work on your profile and pictures. Something else to consider is that there are probably websites and online coaches who might be able to assist with dating.

TASHA: I hadn't thought of that, but I like the sound of the overall plan.

KAILA: If your anxiety doesn't get better, or gets worse, particularly if you continue to have trouble sleeping, you might want to reach out to your primary care physician.

TASHA: Yeah, I will.

KAILA: And lastly, I'm not going anywhere, Tasha. I'm more than willing to talk with you about this again whenever you want. And as noted, I'll follow up with you in the next couple of days.

TASHA: I can't thank you enough, Kaila. I'm glad you came over. I feel so much better, and we have a plan that makes sense.

References

American Psychiatric Association. (2022). Anxiety disorders. In *Diagnostic and statistical manual of mental disorders* (5th ed., text rev.). https://doi.org/10.1176/appi.books.9780890425787.x05_Anxiety _Disorders

Barlow, D. (2002). *Anxiety and its disorders: The nature and treatment of anxiety and panic.* Guilford Press.

Battaglia, M. (2015). Separation anxiety: At the neurobiological crossroads of adaption and illness. *Dialogues in Clinical Neuroscience, 179*(3), 277–285. https://doi.org/10.31887/DCNS.2015.17.3/mbattaglia

Biswas, T., Scott, J. G., Munir, K., Renazho, A. M. N., Rawal, L. B., Baxter, J., & Manmun A. A. (2020). Global variation in the prevalence of suicidal ideation, anxiety and other correlates among adolescents: A population based study of 82 countries. *eClinicalMedicine, 24,* 100395. https://doi.org/10.1016/j.eclinm.2020.100395

Bögels, S. M., Knappe, S., & Clark, L. A. (2013). Adult separation anxiety disorder in DSM-5. *Clinical Psychological Review, 33*(5), 663–674. https://doi.org/10.1016/j.cpr.2013.03.006

Elizur, Y., & Perednik, R. (2003). Prevalence and description of selective mutism in immigrant and native families: A controlled study. *Journal of the American Academy of Child and Adolescent Psychiatry, 42*(12), 1451–1459. https://doi.org/10.1097/00004583 -200312000-00012

Gullone, E. (2000). The development of normal fear: A century of research. *Clinical Psychology Review, 20*(4), 429–451. https://doi.org /10.1016/S0272-7358(99)00034-3

Harvard Medical School. (2007). *National Comorbidity Survey (NCS).* https://www.hcp.med.harvard.edu/ncs/index.php

Kessler, R. C., Petukhova, M., Sampson, N. A., Zaslavsky, A. M., & Wittchen, H.-C. (2012). Twelve-month and lifetime prevalence and lifetime morbid risk of anxiety and mood disorders in the United States. *International Journal of Methods in Psychiatric Research, 21*(3), 169–184. https://doi.org/10.1002/mpr.1359

Muris, P., & Ollendick, T. H. (2015). Children who are anxious in silence: A review on selective mutism, the new anxiety disorder in *DSM-5. Clinical Child and Family Psychology Review, 18,* 151–169. https://doi.org/10.1007/s10567-015-0181-y

National Institute of Mental Health. (n.d.). *I'm so stressed out!* https:// www.nimh.nih.gov/sites/default/files/documents/health/publi cations/so-stressed-out-infographic/so-stressed-out-infographic .pdf

Ruscio, A. M., Hallion, L. S., Lim, C. C. W., Aguilar-Gaxiola, S., Al-Hamzawi, A., Alonso, J., Andrade, L. H., Borges, G., Bromnet, E. J., Bunting, B., de Almeida, J. M. C., Demyttenaere, K., Florescu, S., de Girolamo, G., Gureje, O., Haro, J. M., He, Y., Hinkov, H., Hu, C., de Jonge, P., . . . Scott, K. M. (2017). Cross-sectional comparison of the epidemiology of *DSM-5* generalized anxiety across the globe. *JAMA Psychiatry, 74*(5), 465–475. https://doi.org/10.1001/jamapsychiatry .2017.0056

Santomauro, D. F., Herrera, A. M. M., Shadid, J., Zheng, P., Ashbaugh, C., Pigott, D. M., Abbafati, C., Adolf, C., Amlag, J. O., Aravkin, A. Y., Bang-Jensen, B. L., Bertolacci, G. J., Bloom, S. S., Castellano, R., Castro, E., Chakrabarti, S., Chattopadhyay, J., Cogen, R. M., Collins, J. K., . . . Ferrari, A. J. (2021). Global prevalence and burden of depressive and anxiety disorders in 204 countries and territories in 2020 due to the COVID-19 pandemic. *Lancet, 398*(10312), 1700–1712. https://doi.org/10.1016/S0140-6736(21)02143-7

Strack, J., Lopes, P., Esteves, F., & Fernandez-Berrocal, P. (2017). Must we suffer to succeed? When anxiety boosts motivation and

performance. *Journal of Individual Differences, 38*(2). https://doi.org
/10.1027/1614-0001/a000228

Terlizzi, E. P., & Villarroel, M. A. (2020). *Symptoms of generalized anxiety
disorder among adults: United States, 2019.* NCHS Data Brief No.378.
https://www.cdc.gov/nchs/data/databriefs/db378-H.pdf

Vanin, J. R. (2008). Overview of anxiety and the anxiety disorders. In
Anxiety disorders: Current clinical practice. Humana Press. https://doi
.org/10.1007/978-1-59745-263-2_1

World Health Organization. (2023). *Anxiety disorders.* https://www.who
.int/news-room/fact-sheets/detail/anxiety-disorders

NINE | Anger

NOAH IS A PASSENGER IN A CAR being driven *by his close friend Tyler. The two are in moderately heavy traffic, traveling at around 30 miles per hour, when another driver cuts them off. Almost instantly, Tyler shows signs of road rage. His face turns red, he starts yelling at the other driver, blows his horn repeatedly, begins tailgating, and then speeds up, trying to pull alongside the other car. What does Noah do?*

What Is Anger?

It has been said that the face reflects the inner workings of the body. Phrases like "the purple of anger" and "the pallor of fear" capture how our physical appearance reflects our emotional reactions. Anger is an intense, antagonistic emotional response to frustration, disappointment, emotional hurt, betrayal, injustice, threat, unmet expectations, or failure. One can be angry at another person, a group, a situation, or even oneself. Everyone experiences anger. It is a complex

emotion that is part of the survival response and, as noted below, may at times be adaptive (Callister et al., 2017). But it's the
frequency, intensity, and duration—factors that vary considerably between individuals—that tend to take the greatest toll
(Toledo et al., 2019).

Key Features: Signs and Symptoms

Psychological Symptoms

The following are considered psychological precursors to and
symptoms of anger (Fernandez & Johnson, 2016; Hendricks et al.,
2013):

- Antagonism
- Sense of injustice
- Resentment
- Obsessive thoughts
- Inability to concentrate due to fixation on a person or
  situation
- Reliving a perceived offense or failure
- Dreaming about a perceived offense or failure
- Feeling betrayed
- Feeling wronged
- Holding a grudge

Physical Symptoms

There are numerous responses and physical symptoms associated
with anger. For example, the "purple of anger" noted above reflects
the differential surge of the neurotransmitter that is increasing
gastric processes and blood pressure, which can rise from an average of 120 over 80 to 220 over 130 or even higher. Other physical
signs and symptoms of anger include (Hendricks et al., 2013):

- Clenched fists
- Grinding teeth
- Screaming or shouting
- Increased heart rate (from an average of 60 to 80 beats per minute to as high as 180 beats per minute)
- Dramatic increase in rate of breathing
- Tensing, often unconsciously, of muscles in the neck and face
- Sweating
- Facial discoloration
- Protruding veins
- Clenched jaw

Prevalence of Anger

Factors like temperament, environment, culture, and stress levels influence anger, so it's challenging to accurately determine its frequency. But we all know individuals who both experience and express it frequently. In a national sample of US adults, 7.8% reported having inappropriate, intense, or poorly controlled anger (Okuda et al., 2015). The intensity of anger, which tends to decline with age (Potegal, 2010), can range from mild annoyance to searing rage, sometimes disproportionate to the precipitating event, leading to verbal or physical intimidation or aggression (as displayed by Tyler in the above scenario). In terms of duration, most episodes last less than 30 minutes, though they can last longer when the intensity is higher. Anger commonly arises when other response options or solutions to a problem seem unavailable, becoming a default reaction. Notably, higher socioeconomic status seems to buffer both the intensity and duration of anger (Potegal, 2010).

Negative Impacts of Anger

The expression of anger can have adverse physical and emotional consequences (Marano, 2003). Another, related aspect of anger, one with possible negative consequences, is its suppression, also known as anger-in. Examples of the negative impacts associated with anger (both expressed and held in) are outlined below.

- Anger expression has been associated with increased risk of coronary heart disease events in initially healthy people, as well as a poorer prognosis in those with existing CHD (Chida & Steptoe, 2009).
- Low control of anger has been shown to predict cardiovascular disease in adults aged 25 to 74 years (Haukkala et al., 2010).
- In individuals over age 80 years, experiencing and expressing anger have been found to be more harmful to physical health (increasing inflammation and chronic illness) than sadness (Barlow et al., 2019).
- Conversely, anger-in has been associated with increased pain (Toledo et al., 2019) and peptic ulcers (Chaudhury & Banerjee, 2020).
- An increase in outwardly directed anger and too much suppressed anger (i.e., anger-in) have both been linked with depression (Luutonen, 2007).
- Anger has been associated with sleep disturbances in middle-aged adults (Shin et al., 2005)
- Increased experience and expression of anger have been linked to various anxiety disorders (Hawkins & Cougle, 2011).
- Those who endorsed using psychoactive substances had elevated anger scores compared to nonusers (Laitano et al., 2022),
- Over time, the trait of expressing anger has been associated with an increased risk of diabetes (Mohseni et al., 2023).

- Men with a history of diabetes who frequently experienced strong anger were at particular risk of heart failure (Titova, 2022).
- Compared to healthy participants, those with migraine reported experiencing more intense anger and scored lower on a measure assessing their ability to recognize and manage their emotions (Shaygan et al., 2022)

Positive Effects of Anger?

Clearly there are detriments associated with anger; however, recall that it is embedded in our survival response. So, as mentioned earlier, there are also perceived benefits to anger (Callister et al., 2017; Ratson, 2023). For example, anger has been associated with:

- Discharging physical tension
- Providing motivation or energizing one to make personal changes or find solutions
- Helping one overcome fears
- Recognizing injustices
- Being a visible sign of strength or projected control

Potential E-PFA Recommendations
(Think About Trying This)

What should Noah say to Tyler? What would you say if you were in Noah's position or one similar?

We have somewhat altered the E-PFA intervention approach in this scenario. Given the urgency and intensity of the situation, the processes are more goal-directed, with an added emphasis on safety. Those who are angry can impulsively overreact, so the priority is always safety first!

1) Introduce yourself (if applicable), offer to help, set expectations, de-escalate (if needed).
2) Gather information. (*What happened? What hurts? How bad is it?*) In this scenario, this step can be skipped.
3) Clarify. (*What's the worst part of this?*) This step may or may not be necessary.
4) Provide assistance. (*What do you need right now? How can I help?*) These initial questions can be omitted or rephrased.
   a. *Can Noah use problem-focused assistance?*
   b. *Can Noah use emotion-focused assistance?*
   c. *Can Noah use stress management?*
5) Make a plan. (*Next steps?*)

Introduce Yourself, Offer to Help, Set Expectations, De-escalate

- This situation is unique compared to many of the others in this manual, as it involves physical danger as well as psychological distress. Noah's first job is to do his best to establish a safe environment. This is the moment to be present in a supportive manner while also being assertive about safety, all without escalating Tyler's anger.
- The primary intervention here is de-escalation followed by distraction and refocusing on something other than the anger-provoking situation. Noah should assist Tyler in regaining a sense of control, slowing down the car, and ideally pulling over to a safe place to stop.
- De-escalating an angry person often begins by finding a point of agreement. Noah might say, "I can't believe that guy just cut us off." Using "us" rather than "you" helps reduce the sense of threat and depersonalize the situation.
- Noah might continue, "Tyler, how about slowing down and pulling over? We don't want that guy to get us killed." Doing the

safe thing is also a way of overcoming the actions of the other driver. But if Noah says, "Slow down, you're going to get us killed," he risks being perceived by Tyler as antagonistic, which might fuel the situation, in essence making Noah another target of Tyler's anger. As hard as it may be to believe, sometimes the urge to vent anger temporarily surpasses the instinct to prioritize safety, leading to situations where safety concerns are dismissed.

Gather Information

- Once the car is in a safe location, a brief discussion between Noah and Tyler can ensue. In this scenario, it's pretty clear what happened, and there is no need to review it.
- A direct self-disclosure by Noah might help Tyler vent. For example, Noah could say something like, "I can't believe that guy did that. That's what gets people killed. I don't know whether I was more angry or scared."

Clarify

- After hearing Tyler's response to his statement, a simple paraphrase by Noah could be useful.

Provide Assistance

- In this scenario, the usual questions (*What do you need right now? How can I help?*) and focused responses are used in subtly different forms.

Problem-Focused

- The core issue was Tyler's anger and his excessive speed in trying to catch up to the other driver. Noah should focus on addressing this during de-escalation. It might be helpful for Noah to ask, "What do you need right now to help make your anger go away?"

Emotion-Focused

- Once Tyler has stopped the car, an effective approach would be allowing him to vent and normalizing his anger — *without* reinforcing or validating his dangerous actions.

Stress Management–Focused

- As they continue their drive, distraction is probably the best strategy Noah can use. In other words, it is best not to dwell on the incident. Move on — both physically and psychologically. Shifting the conversation to something unrelated, and even humorous if possible, can help redirect Tyler's attention and diffuse lingering tension.

Make a Plan

- While not essential, Noah might encourage Tyler to anticipate that a similar scenario could arise again in the future and prompt him to think about how he would handle it next time.

E-PFA Dialogue (It Might Sound Like This)

NOAH (TRYING TO REMAIN CALM): Whoa! I don't believe that guy just cut us off!

TYLER: He's driving like an idiot, and I'm not going to let him get away with it.

NOAH: I hear ya, Tyler, but how about slowing down and pulling over? We don't want that guy's bad driving to get us and other people killed. Then he really would be getting the best of us.

TYLER: Exactly. That's why I'm gonna keep letting him know.

NOAH: I know you're a good driver, Tyler, but clearly the same can't be said about this guy. I can't believe he did that. He clearly needs a lesson in driving etiquette, because what he did is what gets people killed. But I don't think now is the time for the driving lesson—and we don't want to give him any more chances to make it worse! I'm trying to decide if I'm more angry or scared.

TYLER: This kind of behavior infuriates me. And who knows, it's possible that he's impaired. That could make it worse.

NOAH: Sounds like you don't want him to get away with this. And I'm with you, but if any part of what you're saying is correct, escalating this could make it worse for all of us.

(Tyler remains silent.)

NOAH: What are you thinking?

TYLER: What's the world coming to?

NOAH: That kind of reckless, selfish move is enough to make anyone furious.

(Tyler slows down and looks to pull over.)

NOAH: Hey, why don't we focus on something more important right now?

TYLER: More important. What could be more important?

NOAH: How about this beautiful night for the concert? I'm curious about the playlist we might hear.

TYLER: You're right. Who needs to get caught up in an angry mess?

NOAH: The way people are driving now, it's probably not the last time we'll run into that kind of careless behavior. So yeah, it's worth thinking ahead—like, what do we do next time it happens? I don't know . . . maybe if we're by ourselves in our car, we could memorize the license plate, pull over, and report it to the police. Just something to keep in mind.

TYLER: Hmm . . . that might be a good plan, Noah.

NOAH: An even better plan for now is to put this aside and enjoy the show.

TYLER: I'm not angry about that!

References

Barlow, M. A., Wrosch, C., Gouin, J.-P., & Kunzmann, U. (2019). Is anger, but not sadness, associated with chronic inflammation and illness in older adulthood? *Psychology and Aging, 34*(3), 330–340. http://dx.doi.org/10.1037/pag0000348

Callister, R. R., Geddes, D., & Gibson, D. F. (2017). When is anger helpful or hurtful? Status and role impact on anger expression and outcomes. *Negotiation and Conflict Management Research, 10*(2), 69–87. https://doi .org/10.1111/ncmr.12090

Chaudhury, P., & Banerjee, U. (2020). Nature of anger, life event stress, conflict and defense mechanism among individuals having peptic ulcer: A comparative study. *Psychological Studies, 65,* 285–295. https://doi.org/10.1007/s12646-020-00559-7

Chida, C., & Steptoe, A. (2009). The association of anger and hostility with future coronary heart disease: A meta-analytic review of prospective evidence. *Journal of the American College of Cardiology, 53*(11), 936–946. https://doi.org/10.1016/j.jacc.2008.11.044

Fernandez, E., & Johnson, S. L. (2016). Anger in psychological disorders: Prevalence, presentation, etiology and prognostic implications. *Clinical Psychology Review, 46,* 124–135. https://doi.org/10.1016/j .cpr.2016.04.012

Haukkala, A., Konttinen, H., Laatikainen, T., Kawachi, I., & Uutela, A. (2010). Hostility, anger control, and anger expression as predictors of cardiovascular disease. *Psychosomatic Medicine, 72*(6), 556–562. https://doi.org/10.1097/PSY.0b013e3181dbab87

Hawkins, K. A., & Cougle, J. R. (2011). Anger problems across the anxiety disorders: Findings from a population-based study. *Depression and Anxiety, 28*(2), 145–152. https://doi.org/10,1002/da.20764

Hendricks, L., Bore, S., Aslinia, D., & Morriss, G. (2013). The effects of anger on the brain and body. *National Forum Journal of Counseling and Addiction, 2*(1), 1–11.

Laitano, H. V., Ely, A., Sordi, A. O., Schuch, F. B., Pechansky, F., Hartmann, T., Hilgert, J. B., Wendland, E. M., Von Dimen, L., Scherer, J. N., Calixto, A. M., Narvaez, J. C. M., Ornell, F., & Kessler, F. H. P. (2022). Anger and substance abuse: A systematic review and meta-analysis. *Brazilian Journal of Psychiatry*, 44(1), 103–110. https://doi.org/10.1590/1516-4446-2020-1133

Luutonen, S. (2007). Anger and depression: Theoretical and clinical considerations. *Nordic Journal of Psychiatry*, 61, 246–251. https://doi.org/10.1080/08039480701414890

Marano, H. E. (2003, July). The downside of anger. *Psychology Today*. https://www.psychologytoday.com/us/articles/200307/the-downside-anger

Mohseni, M., Lindekilde, N., Forget, G., Burns, R. J., Pouwer, F., Schmitz, N., & Deschênes, S. S. (2023). Trait anger, hostility, and the risk of type 2 diabetes and diabetes-related complications: A systematic review of longitudinal studies. *Current Diabetes Reviews*, 19(4), 73–82. https://doi.org/10.2174/1573399818666220329185229

Okuda, M., Picazo, J., Olfson, M., Hasin, D. S., Liu, S.-M., Bernardi, S., & Blanco, C. (2015). Prevalence and correlates of anger in the community: Results from a national survey. *CNS Spectrums*, 20, 130–139. https://doi.org:10.1017/S1092852914000182

Potegal, M. (2010). The temporal dynamics of anger: Phenomena, processes, and perplexities. In M. Potegal, G. Stemmler, & C. Spielberger (Eds.), *International handbook of anger: Constituent and concomitant biological, psychological, and social processes* (pp. 385–401). Springer & Business Media. https://doi.org/10.1007/978-0-387-89676-2_2

Ratson, M. (2023, June). 11 good reasons to get angry. *Psychology Today*. https://www.psychologytoday.com/us/blog/the-wisdom-of-anger/202306/11-good-reasons-to-get-angry

Shaygan, M., Saranjam, E., Faraghi, A., & Mohebbi, Z. (2022). Migraine headaches: The predictive role of anger and emotional intelligence. *International Journal of Community Based Nursing and Midwifery*, 10(1), 74–83. https://doi.org/10.30476/IJCBNM.2021.90552.1706

Shin, C., Kim, J., Yi, H., Lee, H., Lee, J., & Shin, K. (2005). Relationship between trait-anger and sleep disturbances in middle-aged men and women. *Journal of Psychosomatic Research*, 58(2), 183–189. https://doi.org/10.1016/j.jpsychores.2004.07.002

Titova, O. E., Baron, J. A., Michaëlsson, K., & Larsson, S. C. (2022). Anger frequency and cardiovascular morbidity and mortality. *European Heart Journal Open, 2*(4). https://doi.org/10.1093/ehjopen /oeaco50

Toledo, T. A., Hellman, N., Lannon, E. W., Sturycz, C. A., Kuhn, B. L., Payne, M. F., Palit, S., Güereca, Y. M., Shadlow, J. O., & Rhudy, J. L. (2019). Anger inhibition and pain modulation. *Annals of Behavioral Medicine, 53*, 1055–1068. https://doi.org/10.1093/abm/kaz016

TEN | Panic

FAY IS SITTING, RATHER UNCOMFORTABLY, in the middle seat of an exit row in an airplane on a completely full five-and-a-half-hour nonstop flight from San Francisco to Philadelphia. About an hour into the flight, and after the plane experiences some turbulence, she notices that the young man sitting next to her in the window seat, who appears to be in his late 20s, is shaking and lightly perspiring. He turns all the air vents toward himself, begins breathing rapidly, and looks increasingly distressed. He mumbles to himself, "I'm losing it." What should Fay do?

What Is Panic?

Panic is an often unexpected, sudden surge of extreme fear or anxiety that triggers intense physical and emotional reactions, typically peaking in minutes (Baker, 2022). In the scenario above, the passenger seated next to Fay is experiencing a panic attack. According to the *DSM-5-TR* (American Psychiatric Association [APA],

2022), panic attacks are classified under anxiety disorders. But panic can arise from either fear (see Chapter Seven) *or* anxiety (see Chapter Eight). Recall from these earlier chapters that fear involves apprehension and physiological arousal in response to a specific stressor, whereas anxiety involves apprehension and physiological arousal in response to vague or diffuse concerns that are often difficult to identify. Either fear or anxiety can build in a crescendo-like manner that culminates in a panic attack. This buildup may last 5 minutes or more, while the attack itself can continue for several minutes to 10 minutes or longer. The crescendo pattern buildup is a key feature for E-PFA, as it provides a critical window for intervention prior to full-blown panic.

Key Features: Signs and Symptoms

Psychological Symptoms

Panic attacks can be terrifying, often leading the person to believe they are suffocating, having a heart attack or stroke, losing touch with reality, or even dying (APA, 2022). People in the grip of panic frequently feel trapped and may sometimes resort to extreme measures in an attempt to escape. But more commonly, the person feels out of control. Psychologically, panic may present with the following:

- Increased worry (repetitive concern, rumination)
- Fear of losing control
- Fear of dying
- Fear of choking
- Confusion, disorientation
- Difficulty communicating
- Distorted sense of reality, depersonalization
- The need to escape and regain control

Physical Symptoms

A key feature in panic is the sensation of suffocation, driven by shallow, rapid breathing. This type of breathing can lead to hyperventilation, when the body takes in too much oxygen, causing lightheadedness and, in some cases, loss of consciousness. Biologically, panic involves wavelike discharges of the sympathetic (fight-or-flight) nervous system, often resulting in the following:

- Rapid heartbeat
- Trembling or shaking
- Tightness in chest
- Tingling
- Shortness of breath
- Sensations of choking
- Dry mouth
- Dizziness
- Headache
- Sweating
- Paresthesia (numbness or tingling sensations)
- Chills

In some instances, panic can include extreme activation of the parasympathetic nervous system (which controls the processes of resting and digesting), potentially resulting in the following:

- Nausea
- Loss of bladder control
- Loss of bowel control
- Decrease in heart rate and blood pressure
- Fainting

It is not surprising that some investigators describe panic attacks as "false alarms" in which the body's built-in fight-or-flight stress response (see Chapter Six) becomes activated either too often or too intensely (National Institute of Mental Health, 2022).

Individuals who experience repeated panic attacks — and who begin to spend significant time worrying about when the next one might occur, or who alter their behavior to avoid potential triggers (e.g., stopping exercising, avoiding certain places or situations) — may be diagnosed with panic disorder (APA, 2022), a type of anxiety disorder (see Chapter Eight).

Prevalence

In a worldwide survey of close to 143,000 participants, the lifetime prevalence of panic attacks and panic disorder was 13.2% and 12.8%, respectively (de Jonge et al., 2016). These rates are notably higher than those in the United States, where the estimated lifetime prevalence of panic disorder is 4.7% among adults (with rates more than twice as high in females as in males) (Harvard Medical School, 2007), and 2.3% among adolescents (with females slightly more affected than males) (Merikangas et al., 2010). Not unexpectedly, panic disorder has a cultural component (Hinton & Good, 2009; Lewis-Fernández et al., 2010).

Associated Factors or Conditions

It is also important to consider whether other emotional, physical, or behavioral factors may be contributing to a person's experience of panic attacks or panic disorder. These may include co-occurring conditions such as depression (see Chapter Five), anxiety (see Chapter Eight), a history of trauma (see Chapter Eleven), substance use, including alcohol or drug intoxication (see Chapter Thirteen), or physical health issues such as heart disease or thyroid disease. Additional risk factors associated with panic disorder include chronic stress (see Chapter Six), parental over-protection, excessive caffeine consumption, smoking, and limited financial resources (APA, 2022; Moreno-Peral et al., 2014). According to the Cleveland Clinic (2023), having a parent or sibling with panic disorder increases one's risk of developing it by about 40%.

Potential E-PFA Recommendations
(Think About Trying This)

What should Fay say to the young man in the next seat? What would you say if you were in Fay's position or a similar situation?

Given the urgency and high intensity of this situation, our usual intervention approach will be adjusted, similar to the approach proposed for anger in Chapter Nine. The response in this case is more goal-directed, and there is a subtle, but reasonable, safety concern. Those who panic may impulsively overreact.

1) Introduce yourself (if applicable), offer to help, set expectations, de-escalate (if needed).
2) Gather information. (*What happened? What hurts? How bad is it?*)
3) Clarify. (*What's the worst part?*) This step may or may not be necessary.
4) Provide assistance. (*What do you need right now? How can I help?*)
   a. *Can Fay use problem-focused assistance?*
   b. *Can Fay use emotion-focused assistance?*
   c. *Can Fay use stress management?*
5) Make a plan. (*Next steps?*)

Introduce Yourself, Offer to Help, Set Expectations, De-escalate

- Upon noticing the young man's distress, Fay could begin by initiating a conversation. She might say something like, "Forgive me for asking, but are you okay? You look a little distressed." Fay could then introduce herself and ask if he's willing to share his name: "Oh, hi, my name is Fay, what's yours?" (His name is Joshua.)

- The primary intervention in a panic-like situation is often de-escalation, followed by distraction. Initially, it's most important to slow down the breathing pattern before it escalates to hyper-ventilation. Fay might suggest that Joshua and she breathe to-gether in a slower, but not deeper, manner. In the case of a building panic attack, it's essential that Fay present herself as a calm, reassuring presence. Reassurance is especially important since Joshua seems to be beginning to feel a loss of control. Tak-ing a couple of breaths can help them both calm down. Addi-tionally, Fay should be aware that panic attacks are often triggered by anticipation, expectation, and a sense of losing control. There-fore, helping Joshua with distraction and focusing on other things can be especially helpful.

- Psychological "grounding" techniques are also useful in reducing the acute stress associated with anxiety and fear, and especially in mitigating panic. Grounding, a form of distraction (see Chapter Three), could involve Fay encouraging Joshua to focus on an object in the plane or even a sound. She might guide him to sense several different objects for about 15 seconds each, such as how the floor beneath his feet feels, how his arms feel against the armrest, and how his back feels against the seat.

Gather Information

- Either before or immediately after attempting a de-escalation intervention, it can be helpful for Fay to clarify whether Joshua has any medical history that would cause breathing problems or cardiac issues.

- Similarly, Fay should ask Joshua if he is taking any medications that might either contribute to these reactions or, conversely, mitigate his acute distress.
- It's important for Fay to assess, as best she can, whether this is a medical emergency or a psychological one. If it is a medical emergency, she needs to seek immediate medical assistance.
- Otherwise, in this scenario, it is acceptable, but not necessary, for Fay to ask Joshua what seemed to trigger the wave of panic, but only to determine whether there is a stressor that can be removed or altered. In cases of panic, asking the person to focus on the stressor is usually counterproductive, as it will likely accelerate the panic. (*What happened?*)
- Similarly, while it is appropriate for Fay to ask Joshua how he is feeling, it would be unwise to dwell on his symptoms. Focusing too much on what he's experiencing could reinforce his sense that he is losing control. (*What hurts?*)

Clarify

- Here, Fay may offer a paraphrase and clarification to Joshua, something to the effect of, "It sounds like you feel that you're losing control and cannot breathe well." Since Joshua said he was "losing it," it's acceptable for Fay to ask what he meant by that, but merely for clarification, not analysis. (*What's the worst part?*)

Provide Assistance

Problem-Focused

- Fay might ask Joshua what else he thinks he needs. (*What do you need most right now?*)
- If this is truly a medical emergency, she should request medical assistance.
- If not, she can reinforce the grounding techniques.

Emotion-Focused

- Fay could engage Joshua in a conversation about his hobbies, schooling, vacations, the purpose of his trip, or where he grew up—anything to distract him. It's beneficial to focus on something positive.

Stress Management-Focused

- Fay might ask Joshua what he typically does to reduce stress. She could ask him how he has coped with these types of attacks in the past. She can then assess the relevance of his coping strategies in the current situation and encourage him to use them, if appropriate.

Make a Plan

- Before Joshua leaves the plane, Fay can ask him what he might do to help prevent or reduce the intensity of these attacks in the future. Planning helps restore a sense of control.
- She can also ask him who he can follow up with, if needed.
- Fay can remind Joshua that if he is not already receiving psychological or psychiatric support, effective treatments are available for panic.

E-PFA Dialogue (It Might Sound Like This)

FAY: Forgive me for asking, but are you okay?

JOSHUA (BREATHING RAPIDLY): I'm not feeling so good.

FAY (CALMLY): I'm sorry to hear that. Oh, I'm Fay. Would you be okay telling me your name?

JOSHUA *(still breathing rapidly and shaking):* I'm Joshua.

FAY (REMAINING CALM): Hello Joshua, I see that you're breathing rapidly and perspiring. Maybe I can help. When I get really stressed, I find that slowing down my breathing helps. Would you be willing to slow your breathing down with me?

JOSHUA: Yeah . . . okay . . . I know that'll help.

FAY: Okay, let's breathe in through the nose, but not too deeply, and then slowly out through the mouth for a couple of repetitions. And just focus on relaxing as you breathe out.

(fay and Joshua take three breaths together.)

FAY: How's the breathing working for you?

JOSHUA (BREATHING LESS RAPIDLY): It's helping some.

FAY: While we're letting the effects of the breathing settle in, there's something else you can do. If you want, I'd like you to focus your attention for about 15 seconds on how your feet feel on the floor beneath you. Will you do that?

JOSHUA: Just on how it feels?

FAY: That's it. Just on how it feels.

JOSHUA: Okay.

(after 15 seconds.)

FAY: Joshua, now I'd like you to focus for about 15 seconds on how your arms feel against the armrest. Will you do that? You can keep your eyes open or closed, whatever is most comfortable for you. *[Note: Closing one's eyes during airplane turbulence can contribute to dizziness. Keeping one's eyes open and focusing on a spot on the wall can be grounding.]*

JOSHUA (KEEPING HIS EYES OPEN AND APPEARING LESS SHAKY): Okay.

(after 15 seconds.)

FAY: Joshua, the last thing I'd like you to focus on for about 15 seconds is how your back feels against the seat. You good with that?

JOSHUA (SLOWING HIS BREATHING AND CLOSING HIS EYES): Yeah . . . I feel it.

(after 15 seconds.)

FAY: That's good. *(Pauses.)* So, what do you think is going on, Joshua?

JOSHUA: I was feeling like I was suffocating or choking. And I'm a little dizzy. I have had one or two episodes like this in my life that have been described to me as having a panic attack. I'm wondering if that's what's happening now.

FAY: Well, I'm no psychologist, but whatever it is, it sounds scary. Any idea of what might have triggered it?

JOSHUA: Well, I'm not a big fan of flying. It helps when I sit in an aisle seat, but when I booked the flight, there were only window seats and middle seats available. So I took a window seat. This incident started with the turbulence. When the plane started to dip and shake, I looked out the window, and for a second or two I thought for sure I didn't see the wing.

FAY: That sounds pretty frightening. And that's when the feelings started?

JOSHUA: Yeah, I started feeling myself getting hot, starting to sweat, and breathing rapidly. The turbulence stopped . . . for now. The plane is intact. I know the wing is there, but I don't want to look out the window.

FAY: Well, how about closing the window shade for a starter? How's the relaxed breathing working? And are you feeling more grounded in your seat, on the armrest, and on the floor?

JOSHUA: Thanks. It's starting to help. *[Note: Merely engaging in a conversation probably helped by keeping Joshua from focusing on sensations of losing control and anticipating a worse reaction.]*

FAY: What else do you think you might need right now?

JOSHUA (BREATHING MORE REGULARLY): I'm not sure . . .

FAY: Do you need medical assistance?

JOSHUA: No. Thanks. I'm getting better.

FAY: Would it help if we traded seats?

JOSHUA: Umm, thanks. But I think I'm okay staying here. I'm not too eager to try and get up right now.

FAY: Understood. That makes sense. So, is Philadelphia your destination?

JOSHUA: It is. I just passed the journeyman plumber's licensure exam and am pursuing a job opportunity with my uncle who is a master plumber and lives outside of Philly.

FAY: Congratulations. I understand that's a rigorous process.

JOSHUA: Thanks. It is a long and at times tough process. In fact, one of the other times I experienced a panic attack was when I got so stressed out worrying about whether I should become a plumber.

FAY: What have you done in the past to help reduce stress?

JOSHUA: I typically exercise, and I like to play video games. I also play a lot of disc golf—you know using flying discs, like Frisbees, and seeing how many shots it takes to get it into the metal basket that counts as a hole.

FAY: Yeah, I've heard of disc golf. Too bad we can't play it on the plane.

JOSHUA (BREATHING MORE REGULARLY): I'd be up for that!

FAY: You mentioned having these attacks occur a couple of other times. What did you do to cope during these instances?

JOSHUA: I called my mom, who, like you, encouraged me to slow my breathing. She also reassured me that I was going to be okay, and she said that if it ever happens again, I need to repeat to myself that "I am going to be okay" and "This will pass soon" while breathing and finding a quiet space.

FAY: Sounds like really good advice from your mom. And of course you can apply some of it now.

JOSHUA: I couldn't think of those things when the panic started. And once it got going, I was less able to think.

FAY: It's tough to think clearly when we feel out of control. Maybe something to take away is to come up with a plan that uses these strategies if you experience something like this again. That way, you'll feel more in control next time.

JOSHUA: Well, I hope I don't need to use these strategies again, but they sure might help.

FAY: Will you follow up with your mom to let her know what happened, or if you need help?

JOSHUA: I sure will. As soon as I'm off the plane.

FAY: You may already be aware of this, but I've heard there are effective treatments available for panic if you feel you can benefit from them.

JOSHUA (CLOSING HIS EYES AND TAKING A RELAXED, DEEP BREATH): Thanks, Fay.

[Note: Fay's intervention might still have been effective even without the grounding or controlled breathing technique. Simply engaging Joshua in a distracting conversation — about plumbing, where he grew up, his hobbies, or nearly anything unrelated to panic *attacks — could have been enough to help de-escalate and mitigate the situation.]*

References

American Psychiatric Association. (2022). Anxiety disorders. In *Diagnostic and statistical manual of mental disorders* (5th ed., text rev.). https://doi.org/10.1176/appi.books.9780890425787.x05_Anxiety_Disorders

Baker, M. (2022, August). *How long do panic attacks last?* Healthgrades. https://www.healthgrades.com/right-care/anxiety-disorders/how-long-do-panic-attacks-last

Cleveland Clinic. (2023). *Panic attacks and panic disorder.* https://my.clevelandclinic.org/health/diseases/4451-panic-attack-panic-diosrder

de Jonge, P., Roest, A. M., Lim, C. C. W., Florescu, S. E., Bromet, E. J., Stein, D. J., Harris, M., Nakov, V., Caldas-de-Almeida, J. M., Levinson, D., Al-Hamzawi, A. O., Haro, J. M., Viana, M. C., Borges, G., O'Neill, S., de Girolamo, G., Demyttenaere, K., Gureje, O., Iwata, N., . . . Scott, K. M. (2016). Cross-national epidemiology of panic disorder and panic attacks in the World Mental Health Surveys. *Depression and Anxiety, 33*(12), 1155–1177. https://doi.org/10.1002/da.22572

Harvard Medical School. (2007). *National Comorbidity Survey (NCS).* https://www.hcp.med.harvard.edu/ncs/index.php

Hinton, D. E., & Good, B. J. (Eds.). (2009). *Culture and panic disorder.* Stanford University Press.

Lewis-Fernández, R., Hinton, D. E., Laria, A. J., Patterson, E. H., Hofmann, S. G., Craske, M. G., Stein, D. J., Asnaani, A., & Liao, B. (2010). Culture and the anxiety disorders: Recommendations for DSM-V. *Depression and Anxiety, 27*(2), 212–229. https://doi.org/10.1002/da.20647

Merikangas, K. R., He, J-p., Burstein, M., Swanson, S. A., Avenevoli, S., Cui, L., Benjet, C., Georgiades, K., & Swendsen, J. (2010). Lifetime prevalence of mental disorders in U.S. adolescents: Results from the National Comorbidity Survey Replication — Adolescent Supplement (NCS-A). *Journal of the American Academy of Child and Adolescent Psychiatry, 49*(10), 980–989. https://doi.org/10.1016/j.jaac.2010.05.017

Moreno-Peral, P., Conejo-Cerón, S., Motrico, E., Rodríquez-Morejón, A., Fernández, A., García-Campayo, J., Roca, M., Serrano-Blanco, A., Rubio-Valera, M., & Bellón, J. Á. (2014). Risk factors for the onset of panic and generalized anxiety disorders in the general adult population: A systematic review of cohort studies. *Journal of Affective Disorders, 168*(15), 337–348. https://pubmed.ncbi.nlm.nih.gov/25089514/

National Institute of Mental Health. (2022). *Panic disorder: When fear overwhelms.* https://www.nimh.nih.gov/health/publications/panic-disorder-when-fear-overwhelms

ELEVEN | Traumatic Stress

TWENTY-SEVEN-YEAR-OLD MADISON prepares for her weekly seven a.m. bike ride along a 21-mile multiuse trail for biking, running, hiking, and horseback riding. She places her phone and wallet in a pack strapped to the rear rack and her water bottle in a holder on the front of her bike. As with most weekday mornings, especially this early, she is the only one on the trail. Enjoying the scenery, the scent of the morning air, and the sound of chirping birds, she stops to walk her bike through an intersection, about two miles from where she began.

As she enters the clearly marked intersection, she sees a van approaching from her right. Madison pauses to make sure the van stops, which it does. But as she begins to walk again, the van accelerates, hitting the front rim of her bike. Madison is knocked to the ground, sustaining a laceration on her knee, but otherwise physically uninjured. As the van speeds away, she gets a quick glimpse of what appears to be a male driver. Madison screams, "You almost killed me!"

Madison receives physical first aid from a ranger and then reports the incident to the local police. The police indicate that it is unlikely they will be able to find the truck or apprehend the driver. Madison feels disappointed and angry at this discouraging news.

Three weeks later, Madison's knee has healed, but psychological reactions to the incident persist. She awakens every night around three a.m. with nightmares, reliving the accident. She experiences waves of fear whenever she approaches an intersection, whether walking or even driving her car. Equally distressing is her new hypervigilance — constantly scanning every situation for potential threats — and the fact that she feels irritable and easy to anger.

Samantha, a 29-year-old woman and Madison's roommate, has noticed the changes in Madison. While having dinner together one evening at the kitchen table, Madison quietly starts to cry before slamming her water glass onto the table, breaking it and cutting her hand. The cut appears to be a minor laceration. What does Samantha do?

What Is Traumatic Stress?

Traumatic stress results from exposure to a traumatic event, which the *DSM-5-TR* defines as "actual or threatened death, serious injury, or sexual violence" (American Psychiatric Association [APA], 2022). This exposure can occur in several ways: directly experiencing the event, witnessing the event happening to others, learning that it happened to a close family member or friend, or through repeated exposure to the event, as is common with first responders.

Traumatic incidents, including disasters, are deeply embedded in recorded human history. From the eruption of Mount Vesuvius, which buried the city of Pompeii in AD 79, to the Fire of London in 1666, to World War I (1914–1918) and World War II (1939–1945), to the terrorist attacks of September 11, 2001, to Hurricane Katrina in 2005, to the shootings on the Las Vegas strip in 2017, to the COVID-19 pandemic that started in 2020, to the wars in Ukraine and Gaza—these are just a small sample of significant and widespread disasters. Such events are etched into our memories, often receiving national and international attention.

However, it is the recurrent, everyday, smaller-scale traumatic events—such as shootings, fires, accidents, hometown violence, illnesses, and assaults, especially sexual assaults—that can be equally impactful for those who experience them. Consistent with a theme noted throughout this manual, Everly & Lating (2004) suggest that traumatic stress is not solely the result of exposure to the incident, but varies based on what the incident means to the survivors. They assert that traumas that violate core beliefs—such as feelings of trust, safety, order, and justice—can be even more profoundly impactful.

Traumatic Stress and Posttraumatic Stress Disorder

Traumatic stress following a critical incident, also referred to as posttraumatic stress, is an intense response to exposure. Posttraumatic stress disorder (PTSD) is a more severe form of traumatic stress, characterized by symptoms that have persisted at a high intensity and duration, warranting this diagnostic label (APA, 2022).

Key Features: Signs and Symptoms

Symptoms of posttraumatic stress may never reach a threshold that requires a diagnosis of PTSD. Nevertheless, they can be quite disruptive. Symptoms of acute traumatic stress include the following:

- Generalized anxiety (see Chapter Eight)
- Depression (see Chapter Five)
- Specific fears of people, places, or things (see Chapter Seven)
- Intrusive thoughts and memories
- Nightmares
- Avoidance of people, places, or things that trigger memories
- Numbing, dissociation
- Changes in mood, volatility in mood
- Reckless or destructive behavior
- Self-medication with food, drugs, alcohol, or other substances (see Chapter Thirteen)
- Irritability
- Aggressiveness (see Chapter Nine)
- Physical symptoms including heart palpitations, difficulty breathing, or abdominal pains

Most people who go through traumatic events rebound within about 30 days. However, for some people—whether directly or indirectly exposed—symptoms do not resolve and may worsen over time, leading to significant life interference. If symptoms like those listed above persist for three days to one month and cause marked distress and functional impairment, the person may be experiencing what the *DSM-5-TR* refers to as an acute stress disorder (APA, 2022).

If, however, the following combination of symptoms, reactions, and impairments lasts longer than one month, the person may meet the criteria for PTSD (APA, 2022). In a study spanning 24 countries, the 30-day prevalence of trauma-related symptoms consistent with acute stress disorder was 1.4%, while the lifetime prevalence of PTSD was 5.6% (Koenen et al., 2017).

- Intrusive memories (e.g., nightmares and flashbacks about the event)

- Avoidance (either avoiding thinking about the event or avoiding places, people, or activities that remind one of the event)
- Negative changes in thinking and mood (e.g., hopelessness, lack of interest in previously enjoyable activities, difficulty maintaining close relationships)
- Changes in arousal (e.g., irritability or angry outbursts, being easily startled, being on guard for possible danger)

The intensity of these symptoms may vary over time and can be worsened by the stress of daily life or other situations (see Chapter Six). Please note that anyone diagnosed with PTSD should receive formal psychological or psychiatric treatment.

Prevalence of Psychological Trauma and Posttraumatic Stress

According to Ogle and colleagues (2013), approximately 90% of the US population will be exposed to at least one traumatic event during their lifetime. In a global study of nearly 69,000 people across 24 countries, more than 70% reported exposure to at least 1 of 29 types of traumatic events (e.g., witnessing death or serious injury, surviving a life-threatening automobile accident, experiencing a serious illness or injury). Even more troubling, over 30% reported being exposed to four or more such events (Benjet et al., 2016). It seems reasonable to assume that most of these people were ordinary, well-functioning individuals going about their daily lives, many of whom were not emotionally prepared to handle these unpredictable experiences.

Exposure to a traumatic event does not guarantee that a person will develop acute traumatic distress or PTSD. Estimates vary widely, but in general up to 60% of individuals exposed to trauma may develop some symptoms of traumatic distress lasting for about one month. Between 5% and 12% may go on to experience symptoms of PTSD that persist beyond a month. This variability is influenced by an interaction between personal history and the nature of the trauma: Rates tend to be higher among those exposed to combat or sexual assault, for example.

Potential E-PFA Recommendations
(Think About Trying This)

What should Samantha say to Madison? What would you say if you were in Samantha's position or one similar?

The general E-PFA intervention remains fundamentally the same as outlined in Chapter Three, with the added emphasis on attending to physical needs at the outset.

1) Introduce yourself (if applicable), offer to help, set expectations, de-escalate (if needed).
2) Gather information. (*What happened? What hurts? How bad is it?*)
3) Clarify. (*What's the worst part?*) This step may or may not be necessary.
4) Provide assistance. (*What do you need right now? How can I help?*)
    a. *Can Samantha use problem-focused assistance?*
    b. *Can Samantha use emotion-focused assistance?*
    c. *Can Samantha use stress management?*
5) Make a plan. (*Next steps?*)

Introduce Yourself, Offer to Help, Set Expectations, Perform Physical First Aid, De-escalate

- In instances of acute injury, attention should first be given to applying physical first aid, if warranted. Samantha should ask permission to assist Madison, even though she knows her.

- While performing physical first aid, be sure to introduce yourself if you don't know the injured person. This, of course, is unnecessary in the scenario involving Samantha and Madison.
- Samantha might say something like, "Let's patch your hand, then let's talk about what's going on, okay?"
- After attending to Madison's injured hand, Samantha's next step would be to help reduce Madison's current distress. She should maintain a calm, reassuring manner without seeming dismissive of Madison's experience. As she's helping bandage Madison's hand, Samantha might even suggest that Madison take a couple of diaphragmatic breaths along with her.

Gather Information

- Samantha can begin to gain further insight into Madison's challenges while also allowing Madison to express her anger and frustration. She might say, "Madison, I've noticed you haven't quite been yourself since your bike accident. What's been going on?"
- Once Madison describes what happened and how she is feeling, Samantha can try to gauge the severity of Madison's reactions. Remember, determining how bad a crisis reaction is depends both on how much distress Madison expresses, and on the degree to which that distress interferes with her ability to function and carry out what she wants and needs to do.

Clarify

- Here, paraphrasing may be especially useful.
- Samantha can also add her direct observations, especially if Madison seems hesitant or unfocused. Samantha can reflect those observations back to Madison.
- Samantha can ask what the "worst part" of this has been, to provide further clarity both for herself and for Madison, who is

possibly stuck on the thought "He could have killed me." Madison might angrily say, "How could he have done such a thing? And then he just drove away!"

Provide Assistance

- To initiate this phase, Samantha can ask, "What do you need most right now? How can I help?" unless it seems wiser to offer more directive suggestions.

Problem-Focused

- Even if the problem itself cannot be solved, seeking justice is often a course of action that helps survivors of life-threatening incidents cope. It can mitigate the emotional intensity of the experience. In Madison's case, reporting the accident to the police may have been a necessary first step. Most people can accept that accidents happen; what they often find most painful is when injustice follows — such as when the person responsible is not held accountable.

Emotion-Focused

- Samantha could explain to Madison that feeling a bit out of control and angry is a normal response. Acknowledging this helps make the overwhelming, intangible emotions feel more tangible — and therefore more manageable.
- Samantha might also point out that nightmares and hypervigilance are expected and are actually protective in the short run.
- Samantha could mention that Madison seems to be surrendering her well-being to something outside her control (the person in the van who drove off). This could help Madison refocus on the one thing she can control — herself.

Stress Management–Focused

- Stress management incorporates a range of physical and psychological practices designed to help reduce excessive stress. Traumatic stress can be particularly intense. Offering Madison some form of distraction could provide temporary relief, with the understanding that this is likely only a short-term solution until the root cause is addressed.
- Techniques that are especially effective in mitigating the impact of traumatic stress and fostering relaxation include: physical exercise, which helps to release built-up stress (see Chapter Six) and anger (see Chapter Nine); staying busy and distracted (since traumatic stress often involves obsessive thoughts and reliving the event); promoting sleep hygiene (as traumatic stress can interfere with sleep); and meditation and yoga (Loprinzi & Frith, 2019; Sharma, 2014). These methods can be helpful as long as Madison avoids fixating on the accident while trying to relax.
- Samantha can emphasize to Madison the importance of recruiting friends and family (and, if necessary, seeking professional mental health care) for support. In this instance, such support seems imperative.

Make a Plan

- Helping Madison create a plan (*next steps*) for reducing stress and taking back control of her life may be the most important thing Samantha can do. The plan most likely should prioritize obtaining interpersonal support. Given the duration of Madison's symptoms, exploring professional psychological or psychiatric help seems essential. Samantha might reiterate that while nightmares and hypervigilance are common and protective in the short run, they can become debilitating if they persist or intensify.

Thus, obtaining a consultation with a mental health provider would be an important step to consider.

E-PFA Dialogue (It Might Sound Like This)

SAMANTHA: Madison, you're cut and you're bleeding. This looks like it needs attention. May I help you take care of it?

MADISON: I'm sorry I broke the glass; it's really nothing.

SAMANTHA (IN A CALM TONE): Let's patch your hand, then let's talk about what's going on, okay?

MADISON (BECOMING MORE TEARFUL): Okay. Thanks. Listen, I'm not crying because the cut hurts, but I do think I need some help.

SAMANTHA: I hear what you're saying Madison. Give me 30 seconds to go get the first-aid kit. I'll be right back.

MADISON: Thanks.

SAMANTHA (RETURNING WITH THE KIT AND REMAINING CALM): Let's begin by cleaning the area, and then I'll apply a bandage. While I'm doing this, why don't we both take a couple of deep breaths—in through the nose and slowly out through the mouth—to help us relax a bit.

MADISON (DOING THE BREATHING ALONG WITH SAMANTHA AND CRYING LESS): Ahh . . . okay . . . good idea.

SAMANTHA: Is the bandage too tight?

MADISON: No, it's good. Thanks again.

SAMANTHA: You were crying before the glass broke, Madison. And I've noticed that you haven't been yourself since your bike accident three weeks ago. What happened? And what's been happening since?

MADISON: My knee injury after being hit is much better. But I keep having nightmares about the incident, sometimes three or four a week. There are times when I dream about being much more injured, and I hear the van driving away. I'm also increasingly on edge, and I haven't told you this, but I'm hesitant to walk or drive through intersections. There have been multiple instances in the past two weeks where the light changes while I'm driving, I'm slow to move, and the person in the car behind me blows their horn.

SAMANTHA: I appreciate you telling me all this, Madison. I'm also sorry that this is happening to you. Anything else you want to share about how bad things have gotten?

MADISON: I'm starting to be extremely aware of my surroundings. I'm scanning what's around me and I'm waiting for something to happen. I'm alert and on guard. Also, I startle at sounds that never bothered me before, like a door closing — not even slamming. And as you can tell from the broken glass, I'm easily irritable and angry.

SAMANTHA: That sounds really awful, Madison. I didn't realize how bad things were for you. In thinking about it, I noticed the other day that you seemed jumpy when the oven started beeping after it preheated. I didn't make the connection then. I'm sorry.

MADISON: I've been keeping a lot of this to myself, hoping it will go away.

SAMANTHA: It certainly doesn't seem like it's going away. I've recently read that having nightmares and being extra vigilant and having strong startle reactions soon after an incident like yours is not unusual; it's your brain trying to sort out and make sense of what happened and actually trying to protect you. But given the length of time and the intensity of your reactions, it seems like they're becoming more debilitating than protective.

MADISON: That's interesting to know, and I think you might be right.

SAMANTHA: What's been the worst part?

MADISON (BECOMING TEARFUL AGAIN): He could have killed me! Was he trying to kill me? How could he have done such a thing? And then he just drove away! Why?!

SAMANTHA: You seem understandably hurt and angry, Madison.

MADISON: I'm a mess of emotions, and anger is certainly at the forefront.

SAMANTHA: I'm guessing your anger is tied to the fact that the driver didn't stop and isn't being held accountable for what happened.

MADISON: It's unforgivable, totally messed up!

SAMANTHA: I can see how not knowing what really happened or why, and then having no one take responsibility for it would make you feel completely out of control. And with all the emotions you've been dealing with since the accident, it probably just adds to that feeling.

MADISON: I feel as if I have very little, if any, control over anything. And it's awful.

SAMANTHA: Here's something to consider—sometimes being out of control and angry can make those overwhelming feelings more real and tangible, like something you can actually manage.

MADISON: I'm not sure I completely follow what you're saying.

SAMANTHA: What I mean is, you're feeling overwhelmed, which means you're feeling out of control. We need to help you get back some of that sense of control.

MADISON: Oh . . . okay. Any ideas on how to do this?

SAMANTHA: Well, think about it this way. It seems like you're handing over your well-being—something that's so important—to things you can't control, like that careless driver, and the legal system finding justice for you. Do you really want to leave your happiness up to them?

MADISON: Um . . . that's a no! So what do you suggest?

SAMANTHA: That you focus on the one thing you can control.

MADISON: Like . . .

SAMANTHA: Yourself.

MADISON: Ahh.

SAMANTHA: I know what you're going through is intense, and you're dealing with a lot. You've reported the incident to the police and given them as much information as you could. Maybe you can think of some form of distraction, just for a little while, to give you some relief?

MADISON: What are you thinking of?

SAMANTHA: Well, like getting back into exercising. Maybe not biking on the trail for now, but possibly a stationary bike at the gym? You know, I saw that they're starting a new yoga class that meets two nights a week at 6:30 p.m. We could go together. It could be a good way to try to relax and give yourself a break from thinking about what's happened.

MADISON: I like the idea of spending time with you and distracting myself from this as much as possible, but I'm also having difficulties sleeping.

SAMANTHA: There are good sleep hygiene tips on several websites that I'm happy to share with you—things like keeping a regular sleep schedule, making sure your room is dark, having no TV or computer screens on, cutting out caffeine in the evenings, and not hitting the snooze button in the mornings.

MADISON: Hmm . . . send me those websites.

SAMANTHA: Glad to. And please know, Madison, that you're not alone. Consider reaching out to others, like family and friends. I really encourage you to get more interpersonal support as part of your plan for taking back control. Given how long it's been since the accident and how much your reactions seem to be affecting you—especially the nightmares, hypervigilance, and that heightened startle response—it seems that seeking professional mental health support might be an important option.

MADISON: I appreciate your honesty, Samantha. I was actually thinking about this but kept talking myself out of getting outside help. However, if it seems this apparent to you, then I really shouldn't ignore it. I don't want this incident to dictate my life. You're right, I need to take back my control!

SAMANTHA: I'll do all I can to help, including, if you'd like, helping you find a qualified mental health care provider.

MADISON: Thanks.

References

American Psychiatric Association. (2022). Trauma- and stressor-related disorders. In *Diagnostic and statistical manual of mental disorders* (5th ed., text rev.). https://doi.org/10.1176/appi.books .9780890425787.x07_Trauma_and_Stressor-Related_Disorders

Benjet, C., Bormet, E., Karam, E. G., Kessler, R. C., McLaughlin, K. A., Ruscio, A. M., Shahly, V., Stein, D. J., Petukhova, M., Hill, E., Alonso, J., Atwoli, L., Bunting, B., Bruffaerts, R., Caldas-de-Almeida, J. M., de Girolamo, G., Florescu, S., Gurejie, O., Huang, Y., Lepine, J. P., Kawakami, N., Kovess-Masfety, V., Medina-Mora, M. E., Navarro-Mateu, F., Piazza, M., . . . Koenen, K. C. (2016). The epidemiology of traumatic event exposure worldwide: Results from the World Health Survey Consortium. *Psychological Medicine, 46*(2), 327–343. https://doi.org/10.1017/S0033291715001981

Everly, G. S., Jr., & Lating, J. M. (2004). *Personality guided therapy of posttraumatic stress disorder.* American Psychological Association.

Koenen, K. C., Ratanatharathorn, A., Ng, L., McLaughlin, K. A., Bromet, E. J., Stein, D. J., Karam, E. G., Ruscio, A. M., Benjet, C., Scott, K., Atwoli, L., Petukhova, M., Lim, C. C. W., Aguilar-Gaxiola, S., Al-Hamzawi, A., Alonso, J., Bunting, B., Ciutan, M., de Girolamo, G., . . . Kessler, R. C., on behalf of the WHO World Health Survey collaborators. (2017). Posttraumatic stress disorder in the World Mental Health Surveys. *Psychological Medicine, 47*(13), 2260–2274. https://doi.org/10.1017/S0033291717000708

Loprinzi, P. D., & Frith, E. (2019). Protective and therapeutic effects of exercise on stress-induced memory impairment. *Journal of Physiological Sciences, 69*, 1–12. https://doi.org/10.1007/s12576-018-0638-0

Ogle, C., Rubin, G., Bernsten, D., & Siegler, I. (2013). The frequency and impact of exposure to potentially traumatic events over the life course. *Clinical Psychological Science, 1*(4), 426–434. https://doi.org/10.1177/2167702613485076

Sharma, M. (2014). Yoga as an alternative and complementary approach for stress management: A systematic review. *Journal of Evidence-Based Complementary and Alternative Medicine, 19*(1), 59–67. https://doi.org/10.1177/2156587213503344

TWELVE | Eating Disorders

IT'S THE BEGINNING OF SOPHOMORE YEAR *at college for Kendra and Natasha, who roomed together last year with two other women. Now, the two of them share a double room with a bathroom in a different dorm. When Kendra, who spent the summer living and working at a camp for special-needs children, arrives, Natasha is struck by the amount of weight she has lost. After their initial hug, Natasha steps back and asks Kendra if she is okay, noting that she looks so thin. Kendra says she's fine and attributes her weight loss to the awful food at camp.*

Over the first several weeks of the semester, Natasha notices that Kendra frequently skips meals, eats alone, or, when they do eat together, limits herself to salads at lunch and dinner. She also appears to be using an app on her phone to count calories. On days they eat lunch together, Kendra eats quickly, doesn't finish her salad, and then tells Natasha she's going to the library to study. But others have told Natasha that Kendra spends close to two hours daily exercising at the campus fitness center.

Kendra seems increasingly preoccupied and is struggling academically. Her relationship with Natasha is also becoming strained. One evening, as the two of them settle in to watch TV, Natasha orders a pizza from their favorite local place. Kendra seems surprised and distracted, but she puts a slice on her plate. Natasha watches as Kendra subtly removes the cheese and wraps it in a napkin that she folds up and places in the trash can. Natasha turns off the television, looks at Kendra, and says, "We've got to talk."

What Is an Eating Disorder?

Why have we included a chapter on eating disorders in a psychological first aid book? After all, eating is essential for survival, and the brain is responsible for regulating appetite and eating behavior. But many environmental and social factors also influence our eating, and in some cases they can contribute to psychological, social, and even physical dysfunction. As statistics show, disorders of eating are more common than we would like to admit, especially among adolescents, young adults, and even athletes (rates of disordered eating patterns and clinical eating disorders range from 0% to 19% in male athletes and 6% to 45% in female athletes, individuals we typically think of as being in exceptional health) (Bratland-Sanda & Sundgot-Borgen, 2012).

According to the National Institute of Mental Health (2024), eating disorders are serious and potentially fatal illnesses marked by disturbances in eating behaviors (eating too much or too little, or preoccupations with certain types of foods), as well as issues with weight, body image, and related thoughts and emotions. A persistent preoccupation with food, body weight, or body shape may be signs of an underlying eating disorder.

Key Features: Signs, Symptoms, and Other Factors

Psychological Factors

Eating disorders are characterized by persistent disturbances in eating behavior and body weight that substantially impact physical health, emotional well-being, and overall life functioning (American Psychiatric Association [APA], 2022). Their exact causes are unknown; however, psychological factors that are often associated with their development include the following (Bulik et al., 2022):

- Cultural pressure to be thin
- Body dysmorphia (distorted perception of one's body)
- Efforts to exert control, often as a result of being in a highly controlling environment
- Past trauma (see Chapter Eleven)
- Anxiety (see Chapter Eight)
- Stress (see Chapter Six)
- Depression (see Chapter Five)
- Other types of mood disorders
- Social bullying
- Obsessive-compulsive patterns
- Rigid thinking
- Parental pressure to be thin
- History of eating disorders in parents or other family members

Eating disorders are associated with many psychological and social complications, some of which are quite serious or even life-threatening. These include:

- Suicidal thoughts and self-harming behaviors (see Chapter Sixteen)

- Substance misuse (see Chapter Thirteen)
- Work or school problems
- Social isolation
- Severe depression (see Chapter Five)

Physical Symptoms

Eating disorders can lead to physical complications and medical conditions, including:

- Low red blood cell count (anemia)
- Chronic fatigue
- Kidney stones
- Heart problems (e.g., arrhythmias, slow heart rate, mitral valve prolapse, heart failure, death)
- Low blood pressure
- Electrolyte imbalance (e.g., low calcium, low phosphorous, low magnesium)
- Bloating
- Constipation
- Lack of menstrual periods in women
- Low testosterone in men
- Bone density loss (osteoporosis)
- Muscle loss
- Disorders of the esophagus, stomach, and intestines

Prevalence of Eating Disorders

Eating disorders occur across culturally and socially diverse groups. In 2019, the global number of diagnosed eating disorders was estimated at around 55.5 million (Santomauro et al., 2021). These disorders most often develop in adolescence or young adulthood. Notably, the estimated lifetime prevalence of eating disorders worldwide among people age 30 and younger ranges from 5.5% to 17.9% in women and from 0.6% to 2.4% in men (Silén & Keski-Rahkonen, 2022). Another study found that around 22% of children and adolescents worldwide exhibit some form of disordered eating (López-Gil et al., 2023). During the COVID-19 pandemic, the incidence of eating disorders in the United States rose an estimated 15.3% in 2020 compared to prepandemic levels in 2019 (Taquet et al., 2021).

According to the National Eating Disorders Association (n.d.), an estimated 30 million Americans (20 million women and 10 million men) will struggle with an eating disorder at some point during their lifetime. Although eating disorders can affect people of any age, gender, body weight, or racial/ethnic background, recent attention in the United States has highlighted their prevalence and impact within specific populations, including athletes (as noted above), members of the LGBTQ+ community, and people of color (Flatt et al., 2021; Parker & Harriger, 2020; Simone et al., 2022).

Types of Eating Disorders

The following are the four most common eating disorders outlined in the *DSM-5-TR* (APA, 2022).

Anorexia Nervosa

Anorexia nervosa, commonly referred to as anorexia, is a condition in which individuals either avoid food, restrict their intake, or eat only small amounts of a few select foods. People with anorexia typically have a distorted body image and an irrational fear of gaining weight, and their self-esteem is tied closely to their weight. As a result, it is not unusual for them to weigh themselves frequently, and even when extremely underweight they may still perceive themselves as overweight and continue pursuing weight loss. The lifetime global prevalence of anorexia nervosa among those age 30 and younger is estimated at 0.8–6.3% in women and 0.1–0.3% in men (Silén & Keski-Rohkonen, 2022).

There are two types of anorexia:

1) restrictive, in which the amount of food consumed is severely limited, and weight loss is primarily accomplished through dieting, fasting, and/or exercising;
2) binge-purge, in which food intake is also restricted, but episodes of consuming large amounts of food are followed by efforts to eliminate the food, such as self-induced vomiting or misuse of laxatives, enemas, or diuretics (to help eliminate water weight).

Prolonged anorexia has been linked to structural and functional brain changes (Kawakami et al., 2022). The consequences of anorexia can be severe, even fatal. People with anorexia face a fivefold increased mortality risk (van Eeden et al., 2021). In a large US study examining suicide attempts among those with lifetime anorexia, 15.7% of individuals with restricting anorexia and 44.1% of those with the binge-purge type had attempted suicide (Udo et al., 2019).

Bulimia Nervosa

Bulimia nervosa, commonly referred to as bulimia, is characterized by recurrent episodes of binge eating, in which individuals consume unusually large amounts of food (typically within a two-hour window) and feel a lack of control over their eating (APA, 2022). This overeating, often done in secrecy, is typically followed by feelings of guilt, shame, or fear of weight gain, which leads individuals to seek ways to eliminate the ingested calories through purging. Common purging behaviors include self-induced vomiting (the most frequent method), overexercising, refusing to eat, and misuse of laxatives or diuretics. People with bulimia nervosa typically have body weight ranging from slightly underweight to normal or overweight. According to the *DSM-5-TR* (APA, 2022), bingeing and purging occur at least once a week for a minimum of three months. The worldwide prevalence of bulimia nervosa among those age 30 and under is estimated to be 0.8–2.6% in women and 0.1–0.2% in men (Silén & Keski-Rahkonen, 2022).

Some of the unique features of bulimia nervosa include:

- Worn tooth enamel (from excessive vomiting)
- Gastrointestinal problems
- Damaged taste receptors
- Intestinal irritation from laxative use
- Severe dehydration
- Swollen and sore throat
- Nutritional deficiencies
- Esophageal tears (these are rare)
- Cardiac problems (also rare)

Similar to anorexia, individuals with bulimia face a fivefold increased mortality risk (van Eeden et al., 2021). In the same large US study referenced earlier, 31.4% of those with bulimia nervosa have made a suicide attempt (Udo et al., 2019).

Binge-Eating Disorder

Binge-eating disorder (BED) is a condition in which individuals, like those with bulimia nervosa, experience a loss of control over their eating and have frequent episodes of consuming unusually large quantities of food. These episodes are often marked by eating rapidly, eating until uncomfortably full, eating large amounts when not physically hungry, or eating alone due to embarrassment. They are typically followed by feelings of shame, guilt, or self-disgust (APA, 2022). As with bulimia, this pattern of binge eating occurs at least once a week for a minimum of three months.

Unlike bulimia, however, these episodes are not followed by purging behaviors such as vomiting, excessive exercise, or fasting. Partly because of this lack of compensatory behavior, symptoms can persist for years and go unnoticed or underreported to health care professionals. In the United States, BED affects an estimated 3.5% of women and 2% of men and is considered to impact 30–40% of individuals seeking weight loss treatment (National Alliance for Eating Disorders, 2024). Lifetime worldwide prevalence of BED is estimated to be 0.2–6.1% in adolescents, 0.6–1.8% in adult women, and 0.3–0.7% in adult men (Keski-Rahkonen, 2021).

Some of the associated consequences of binge eating include:

- Obesity
- Metabolic disturbances
- Type 2 diabetes
- Hypertension
- Social adjustment problems

As with other eating disorders, binge-eating disorder is associated with increased mortality—approaching twice the expected rate. Moreover, 94% of a sample of individuals with BED report lifetime mental health issues, including substance use (68%) (see Chapter Thirteen); anxiety (59%) (see Chapter Eight); and depression (70%) (see Chapter Five). Up to 23% reported attempting suicide (Keski-Rahkonen, 2021; Udo et al., 2019) (see Chapter Sixteen).

Avoidant/Restrictive Food Intake Disorder

Avoidant/restrictive food intake disorder (ARFID), previously known as selective eating disorder, is a condition where people avoid or limit the amount or type of food they eat. Unlike anorexia nervosa, the failure to meet dietary needs is not due to body image concerns, fear of weight gain, medical issues, or cultural reasons. Instead, ARFID is related to the following (APA, 2022):

- Dislike and avoidance of a food's sensory characteristics (e.g., appearance, smell, texture, taste, temperature), which is common in individuals with autism
- Concern or worry about adverse experiences after eating, such as choking or vomiting
- Lack of interest in food

ARFID is associated with substantial weight loss, caloric and other nutritional deficiencies, adversely impacted growth and development, impaired social functioning, and, in more severe cases, the need for tube feeding or oral nutritional supplements (APA, 2022). ARFID may begin as early as infancy and can persist into adulthood. Yet it is more than just a childhood phase of "picky eating," because it can become progressively worse. Since it is a newer diagnosis compared to other eating disorders, there is limited information on its prevalence. A recent study (Van Buuren et al., 2023) found that 1.98% of adolescents between ages 11 and 19 had possible ARFID, with females being 1.7 times more likely than males to have the condition. Interestingly, in a study of individuals with ARFID, 12% developed body image concerns that warranted a diagnostic change to anorexia nervosa (Norris et al., 2014). A study of children and adolescents with ARFID found that 8% reported current suicidal ideation, and 14% reported lifetime ideation (Kambanis et al., 2020).

Potential E-PFA Recommendations
(Think About Trying This)

What can Natasha do to assist her friend Kendra, who appears to be struggling with a serious eating disorder, as evidenced by weight loss, poor nutrition, and declining academic performance? What would you say if you were in Nathasa's position or one similar?

Let's consider the situation through the five-phase E-PFA lens. Listed below are potential E-PFA interventions that Natasha might use to support Kendra.

It's essential to keep in mind that Natasha's intervention is a psychological Band-Aid. It's not intended to "fix" or "cure" Kendra but to assist her in getting the help she needs. The following recommendations offer general guidelines and considerations for mitigating distress and guiding Kendra to the next level of care.

The general E-PFA intervention remains fundamentally the same as we have seen in other chapters:

1) Introduce yourself (if applicable), offer to help, set expectations, de-escalate (if needed).
2) Gather information. (*What happened? What hurts? How bad is it?*)
3) Clarify. (*What's the worst part?*)
4) Provide assistance. (*What do you need right now? How can I help?*)
   a. *Can Natasha use problem-focused assistance?*
   b. *Can Natasha use emotion-focused assistance?*
   c. *Can Natasha use stress management?*
5) Make a plan. (*Next steps?*)

Introduce Yourself, Offer to Help, Set Expectations

- PFA begins with showing up and expressing a calm, nonconfrontational concern. Natasha can expect Kendra to initially deny there is any problem. Eating disorders are considered variations on compulsive disorders, which often come with rigid, narrow-minded thinking, denial as a defense mechanism, and some degree of shame. Therefore, Natasha should avoid confrontation or argument. Rather, she should calmly share her observations and concerns, sticking to the facts as she's observed them.

Gather Information

- Natasha should encourage Kendra to talk about what she is experiencing, using questions like, "What's going on?" and "When did you start dieting like this?" (*What happened?*)
- Once Kendra begins to share her thoughts, Natasha might ask, "What prompted you to start dieting like this?" (*What hurts?*)
- Natasha should try to assess the overall severity and urgency of the situation through questions like, "How long has this been going on?" and "How much weight have you lost?" (*How bad is it?*)

Clarify

- The clarification phase usually begins with a paraphrase or recap of what Natasha heard regarding when the dieting started and the motivation behind it.
- It's important that Natasha remain nonjudgmental in her approach.
- Asking "What's the worst part?" may not be useful at this stage, as Kendra is likely to deny or minimize the problem initially.

Provide Assistance

- Natasha can start by asking, "What do you need most right now?" and "How can I help?" She can also consider using the more directive options outlined below.

Problem-Focused

- The problem is the eating disorder, and the goal is to help Kendra seek professional assistance. Since eating disorders are classified as psychiatric disorders, Natasha should treat this as a medical emergency.

- As mentioned, Natasha should expect Kendra to initially deny there's a problem. Therefore, a calm, nonargumentative response where Natasha simply notes what she has observed may be her best course of action. The dramatic weight loss, persistent sadness, poor nutrition, and failing academics provide persuasive evidence of a problem, without even attaching a label to it.

Emotion-Focused

- Emotion-focused PFA when addressing someone with an eating disorder involves avoiding argumentation, confrontation, or anything else that might provoke denial and cause the person to walk away. In this instance, Natasha could simply allow Kendra to vent.

Stress Management–Focused

- Stress management–focused intervention will involve Natasha helping Kendra come up with alternative ways of coping with stress, particularly if Kendra reveals that her eating behaviors are a means of managing stress, a lack of control, bullying, or other factors that she believes are associated with her symptoms.

Make a Plan

- As mentioned above, an eating disorder should be considered a medical emergency. Natasha should act accordingly, meaning her goal is to support Kendra in seeking treatment. While this may not require calling 911 or accessing emergency medical support, it will likely entail developing a concrete plan for obtaining assistance—which Kendra may initially resist or delay. (*Next steps?*)

E-PFA Dialogue (It Might Sound Like This)

NATASHA (CALMLY): Kendra, I'm concerned about you. What's going on?

KENDRA: What do you mean? What are you concerned about?

NATASHA: I just saw you take the cheese off the slice of pizza, put it in a napkin, and throw it away.

KENDRA: Oh, you saw that? It was just a bad slice of pizza, that's it.

NATASHA: A bad slice of pizza? Is there such a thing?

KENDRA: It just didn't taste right. It's no big deal.

NATASHA (CALMLY): Kendra, it's me. What's going on?

KENDRA: Okay . . . I've started a low-carb diet, and pizza is not a part of it.

NATASHA: When did you start dieting like this?

KENDRA: At the camp I was working at over the summer.

NATASHA: What prompted you to start this diet?

KENDRA: As I mentioned when I first got back to campus, the food there was awful, so it made sense to try and eat differently. That's it!

NATASHA (STILL CALMLY): Kendra, I hear you saying that you started this diet recently and it was because the food at the summer camp was bad, but I think there's possibly more going on with you. You've been skipping meals, you seem to be using a phone app to track your calories, and you have lost a noticeable amount of weight. I'm really worried that you might be struggling with something more serious.

KENDRA: I appreciate the concern, Natasha, but I'm just trying to eat healthier.

NATASHA: I understand that, and I hope you can appreciate that everything I'm saying is based solely on my genuine concern for you.

KENDRA: So, is there more?

NATASHA: Well, others who know both of us have told me that they've seen you at the fitness center running on a treadmill for hours. Also, you shared with me that your grades so far this semester are not good. And let's be real, there's been a strain in our relationship for the past several weeks that's never been there before.

Listen, I understand that you want to eat healthy, but it seems that you might be developing an unhealthy relationship with food and your body. This can be really hard, and particularly hard to handle by yourself. Again, Kendra, I just want to make sure you're okay.

KENDRA: I'm working to handle this. I'm not sure I need any help.

NATASHA: I hear you, and I respect that you are working on handling this on your own. But, Kendra, the dramatic weight loss, poor nutrition, and your mood change suggest that what you're doing isn't working. And I will feel awful if it gets worse and I don't offer to help you get the support that I truly believe you need.

KENDRA (after a 30-second pause): Wow! Has it been this apparent? I had no idea.

NATASHA: Since you've been back, it's become increasingly obvious. So, yeah, it's that apparent.

KENDRA: It's just been hard. I feel such pressure to look more like my very thin sister, and once I began losing weight, and then more weight over the summer, I became more and more focused on keeping it going, whether by dieting or exercising. I'm feeling more and more stressed and out of control.

NATASHA: I can only imagine how tough all of this is for you. And I admire you sharing this with me. I'm here for you. You're not alone in this.

KENDRA: Thanks, Nathasha.

NATASHA: We need to come up together with a plan to find other, alternative ways, to help you feel more in control of what's going on with your eating, mood, and exercising.

KENDRA: What are you thinking?

NATAHSA: I sincerely believe that what you currently need is treatment from a health care professional. So, how about if tomorrow we plan on contacting a professional to get you seen as soon as possible?

KENDRA: Whew . . . this is a lot to handle. Let me think about it and sleep on it. (20-second pause.) But you're probably right.

NATAHSA: I'm with you every step of the way. Promise me that we'll talk first thing tomorrow.

KENDRA: I promise.

References

American Psychiatric Association. (2022). Feeding and eating disorders. In *Diagnostic and statistical manual of mental disorders* (5th ed., text rev.). https://doi.org/10.1176/appi.books.9780890425787.x10_Feeding_and_Eating_Disorders

Bratland-Sanda, S., & Sundgot-Borgen, J. (2012). Eating disorders in athletes: Overview of prevalence, risk factors and recommendations for prevention and treatment. *European Journal of Sport Science, 13*(5), 499–508. https://doi.org/10.1080/17461391.2012.740504

Bulik, C. M., Colemena, J. R. I., Hardaway, J. A., Breithaupt, L., Watson, H. J., Bryant, C. D., & Breen, G. (2022). Genetics and neurobiology of

eating disorders. *Nature Neuroscience, 25,* 543–554. https://doi.org/10
.1038/s41593-022-01071-z

Flatt, R. E., Thorton, L. M., Fitzsimmons-Craft, E. E., Balantekin, K. N.,
Smolar, L., Mysko, C., Wilfley, D. E., Taylor, C. B., DeFreese, J. D.,
Bardone-Cone, A. M., & Bulik, C. M. (2021). Comparing eating
disorder characteristics and treatment in self-identified competitive
athletes and non-athletes form the National Eating Disorders
Association online screening tool. *International Journal of Eating
Disorders, 54*(3), 363–375. https://doi.org/10.1002/eat.23415

Kambanis, P. E., Kuhnle, M. C., Wons, Q. B., Jo, J. H., Keshishian, A. C.,
Hauser, K., Becker, K. R., Franko, D. L., Misra, M., Micali, N.,
Lawson, E. A., Eddy, K. T., & Thomas, J. J. (2020). Prevalence and
correlates of psychiatric comorbidities in children and adolescents
with full and subthreshold avoidant/restrictive food intake disorder. *International Journal of Eating Disorders, 53*(2), 256–265. https://
doi.org/10.1002/eat.23191

Kawakami, I., Iritani, S., Riku, Y., Umeda, K., Takase, M., Ikeda, K.,
Nizato, K., Arai, T., Yoshida, M., Oshima, K., & Hasegawa, M. (2022).
Neuropathological investigation of patients with prolonged
anorexia nervosa. *Psychiatry and Clinical Neurosciences, 76,* 187–194.
https://doi.org/10.1111/pcn.13340

Keski-Rahkonen, A. (2021). Epidemiology of binge eating disorder:
Prevalence, course, comorbidity, and risk factors. *Current Opinions
in Psychiatry, 34,* 525–531. https://doi.org/10.1097/YCO.000000
0000000750

López-Gil, J. F., García-Hermoso, A., Smith, L., Firth, J., Trott, M.,
Mesas, A. E., Jiménez-López, E., Gutiérrez-Espinosa, H., Tárraga-
López, P. J., & Victoria-Montesinos, D. (2023). Global proportion of
disordered eating in children and adolescents. *JAMA Pediatrics,
177*(4), 363–372. https://doi.org/10.1001/jamapediatrics.2022.5848

National Alliance for Eating Disorders (2024). Eating disorder
statistics: An updated view for 2024. https://www.alliancefore
atingdisorders.com/eating-disorder-statistics-an-updated-view-for
-2024

National Eating Disorders Association (NEDA). (n.d.). https://www
.nationaleatingdisorders.org

National Institute of Mental Health. (2024). *Eating disorders.* https://
www.nimh.nih.gov/health/topics/eating-disorders

Norris, M. L., Robinson, A., Obeid, N., Harrison, M., Spettigue, W., &
Henderson, K. (2014). Exploring avoidant/restrictive food intake

disorder in eating disordered patients: A descriptive study. *International Journal of Eating Disorders, 47*(5), 495–499. https://doi.org/10.1002/eat.22217

Parker, L. L., & Harriger, J. A. (2020). Eating disorders and disordered eating behaviors in the LGBT population: A review of the literature. *Journal of Eating Disorders, 8*, 51. https://doi.org/10.1186/s40337-020-00327-y

Santomauro, D. F., Melen, S., Mitchison, D., Vos, T., Whiteford, H., & Ferrari, A. J. (2021). The hidden burden of eating disorders: An extension of estimates from the Global Burden of Disease Study 2019. *Lancet Psychiatry, 8*(4), 320–328. https://doi.org/10.1016/S2215-0366(21)00040-7

Silén, Y., & Keski-Rahkonen, A. (2022). Worldwide prevalence of DSM-5 eating disorders among young people. *Current Opinion in Psychiatry, 35*(6), 362–371. https://doi.org/10.1097/YCO.0000000000000818

Simone, M., Telke, S., Anderson, L. M., Eisenberg, M., & Neumark-Sztainer, D. (2022). Ethnic/racial and gender differences in disordered eating behavior prevalence trajectories among women and men from adolescence to adulthood. *Social Science and Medicine, 294.* https://doi.org/10.1016/j.socscimed.2022.114720

Taquet, M., Geddes, J. R., Luciano, S., & Harrison, P. J. (2021). Incidence and outcomes of eating disorders during the COVID-19 pandemic. *British Journal of Psychiatry, 220*(5), 262–264. https://doi.org/10.1192/bjp.2021.105

Udo, T., Bitley, S., & Grilo, C. M. (2019). Suicide attempts in US adults with lifetime DSM-5 eating disorders. *BMC Medicine, 17*, 120. https://doi.org/10.1186/s12916-019-1352-3

Van Buuren, L., Fleming, C. A. K., Hay, P., Bussey, K., Trompeter, N., Lonergan, A., & Mitchison, D. (2023). The prevalence and burden of avoidant/restrictive food intake disorder (ARFID) in a general adolescent population. *Journal of Eating Disorders, 11*, 104. https://doi.org/10.1186/s40337-023-00831-x

van Eeden, A. E., van Hoeken, D., & Hoek, H. W. (2021). Incidence, prevalence and mortality of anorexia nervosa and bulimia nervosa. *Current Opinion in Psychiatry, 34*, 515–524. https://doi.org/10.1097/YCO.0000000000000739

THIRTEEN | Intoxication

MEGAN, A 24-YEAR-OLD RECEPTIONIST *at a presti-gious law firm, texts her friend Daria around nine a.m. saying she really needs to talk. After Daria agrees, Megan suggests they meet after work at a local bar they frequently visit for Friday happy hour. Daria, sensing the urgency, tries to make sure to leave work on time but ends up running late and texts Megan that she'll be about 30 minutes behind. Megan does not reply.*

When Daria arrives, she sees Megan at the bar with three empty wine glasses and two empty shot glasses in front of her. As Daria walks toward her, Megan orders two more shots of vodka. Daria asks what's going on. Megan, her voice loud and words slurred, says, "I think I have a drinking problem." She laughs and lays her head on the bar.

Daria is stunned—she has known Megan for two years and has never seen her drink more than two drinks, let alone appear this intoxicated. Megan then reveals that her fiancé ended their relationship after admitting he had been seeing someone else and now wants to be with that person. Megan downs another shot, looks at Daria, and says, "I need help." What does Daria do?

What Is Intoxication?

According to the *Merriam-Webster* online dictionary (n.d.), intoxication is "the condition of having physical or mental control markedly diminished by the effects of alcohol or drugs." Technically, intoxication represents an altered state of consciousness. The symptoms and severity of intoxication can vary based on factors such as body weight, whether there's food in one's stomach, and the person's history with or tolerance to the substance. From a physiological standpoint, alcohol intoxication occurs when alcohol enters the bloodstream faster than the liver can metabolize it. In the case of other substances, intoxication results from their direct effects on the brain's neural circuitry, causing consciousness-altering effects.

Reasons for using substances that cause intoxication are numerous and varied but may include:

- Relaxation
- Desire to experience an altered state of consciousness
- Mood enhancement
- Removal of inhibition
- Thrill-seeking
- Self-medication after an adverse experience
- Social pressure
- Coping with general stress
- Addiction, which is a self-sustaining process

In this chapter, our E-PFA approach addresses intoxication as a general process without focusing on the specific substance involved. In addition, for reference, we provide substance-specific information after the example dialogue.

Key Features: Signs and Symptoms

Psychological Symptoms

Psychologically, intoxication affects both the cognitive (thinking) and the affective (emotional) domains of behavior. To make a sweeping generalization, intoxication has a disinhibiting effect. Intoxicants interfere with normal communication between the prefrontal cortex, which is responsible for rational thought and self-control, and the subcortical structures of the limbic system, which are responsible for emotions and the fight-or-flight survival mechanisms (see Chapters Six and Seven). Some intoxicants also disrupt the normal function of certain neurotransmitters such as dopamine and serotonin.

The effects of intoxicants may include, but are not limited to, the following:

- Short-term effects
  - Euphoria
  - Reduced inhibitions
  - Rapid mood swings
  - Aggression
  - Impaired judgment
  - Inability to understand the consequences of one's actions
  - Panic (see Chapter Ten)
  - Paranoia (see Chapter Seventeen)
  - Inability to follow instructions
  - Memory loss
  - Sadness (see Chapter Five)
  - Suicidal ideation (see Chapter Sixteen)

- Long-term effects
  - Depression (see Chapter Five)
  - Cognitive decline
  - Anxiety (see Chapter Eight)
  - Inclinations toward irritability, violence, or anger (see Chapter Nine)

Physical Symptoms

Physically, intoxicants can affect both fine and gross motor systems, the gastrointestinal system, the respiratory system, and the cardiovascular system. The effects of intoxicants may include, but are not limited to, the following:

- Impaired motor coordination
- Memory distortion
- Heart arrythmias
- Impaired speech
- Nausea, vomiting
- Difficulty walking
- Slowed reaction times
- Interference with hand-eye coordination
- Rapid changes in blood pressure
- Loss of consciousness
- Seizures
- Poisoning

Potential E-PFA Recommendations
(Think About Trying This)

What can Megan's friend Daria do to assist Megan during what appears to be an acute episode of intoxication? What would you say or do if you were in Daria's position or one similar?

Let's look at this situation through the five-phase E-PFA lens we have used in other chapters. Daria's primary focus should be on Megan's safety and well-being in the current moment. Remember, this intervention is a psychological Band-Aid. It is not meant to resolve Megan's relationship challenges or even address what might be an emerging pattern of self-medication (though that seems unlikely given Megan's history). The goal is to provide immediate support and ensure Megan gets the help she needs now, with follow-up care considered afterward, if appropriate.

The general E-PFA intervention is far more targeted when dealing with a situation like this one. As with the cases of anger (see Chapter Nine) and panic (see Chapter Ten), safety for both the intoxicated person and the person trying to help are always concerns.

1) Introduce yourself (if applicable), offer to help, set expectations, de-escalate (if needed).
2) Gather information. (*What happened? What hurts? How bad is it?*) This phase targets the intoxication and what led to it.
3) Clarify. (*What's the worst part?*) This phase focuses on clarifying the source and degree of intoxication.
4) Provide assistance. (*What do you need right now? How can I help?*) These questions are unnecessary here.
   a. *Can Daria use problem-focused assistance?*
   b. *Can Daria use emotion-focused assistance?*
   c. *Can Daria use stress management?*
5) Make a plan. (*Next steps?*)

Introduce Yourself, Offer to Help, Set Expectations, De-escalate

- Intervention in this instance is occurring in a public place, which presents challenges when assisting someone as intoxicated as Megan. There are elements of the environment that Daria cannot control and which could pose a risk of escalation or otherwise compromise Megan's safety.

- Daria's safety is also a consideration as intoxicated people often are disinhibited, may act impulsively, and can behave without understanding the consequences of their actions.
- Another consideration is that, given the amount of alcohol consumed in a short period of time, Megan's level of intoxication will likely worsen before it improves. This presents three likely challenges: (1) Megan may soon be unable to walk unassisted, (2) she may lose consciousness, and (3) she may deny needing assistance. That said, in this scenario, Megan's statement—"I need help"—provides a potential opening. While she may be referring to the emotional devastation of losing her fiancé, Daria can interpret it as an opportunity to assist Megan in her intoxicated state.
- As always, E-PFA begins with "showing up" and expressing a calm, nonconfrontational concern. In this case, the two need to leave the bar and get Megan home.

Gather Information

- Megan has given Daria the information she needs to act. Daria knows Megan is highly intoxicated, and she knows the source of the intoxication is at least alcohol.
- The existence of other substances that interact with alcohol could turn this scenario into a life-threatening medical emergency, so it's important for Daria to ask what other substances or medications might also be affecting Megan. Megan has had three glasses of wine and three shots of vodka. No other substances were reported. A 125-pound female who consumes this quantity of alcohol within one hour would likely have a blood alcohol content (BAC) significantly above the legal limit, potentially around 0.15%, placing her in a state of substantial intoxication. (For context, one

shot of distilled spirits equals about 5 ounces of wine or 12 ounces of beer; see the additional section on alcohol, below, for more about what constitutes a serving of alcohol. For a 125-pound woman, each drink can raise BAC by roughly 0.035% per hour, while for a 180-pound man, it's about 0.02%. Blood alcohol levels typically decline by about 0.015% per hour due to liver metabolism.)

- If Daria determines that Megan is safe, she can choose one of two approaches: She can discuss Megan's stressful relationship at the bar and then transition to a more in-depth conversation at Megan's home, or she can act immediately to get Megan home, ensuring her safety first, and then talk about the relationship. Given the amount of alcohol consumed, the longer Daria waits to help Megan with the immediate problem (her intoxication), the more difficult it will be for her to assist Megan.

- Daria should quickly assess the severity and urgency (*How bad?*) of Megan's intoxication, which requires immediate attention.

Clarify

- The clarification phase begins with Daria paraphrasing or recapping what she has heard about Megan's consumption of alcohol and any other substances. While Daria could express sympathy for the behavior of Megan's fiancé, she should quickly shift focus to the alcohol as the more pressing concern in the moment.

Provide Assistance

- Here are some options for Daria to consider.

Problem-Focused

- The goal is to get Megan to a safe quiet place with few or no additional stressors — most likely her home.

- Daria should be firm in refusing to allow Megan to drink more.
- Daria should make sure the bill gets paid.
- Daria should accompany Megan home.
- Daria should make sure Megan remains sitting up if she is awake. If Megan passes out, placing her on her side can reduce the risk of choking.
- Daria should not provide coffee, other beverages, or food as these can increase the risk of choking. Sips of water are generally safe if Megan is thirsty.
- Cold showers or exercise will not lessen intoxication and may increase the risk of physical injury.
- Daria should monitor Megan's breathing. Central nervous system depressants such as alcohol can suppress breathing and heart function, and in some cases—especially when combined with other substances—can be fatal.
- When in doubt, Daria should call for emergency medical support.

Emotion-Focused

- Emotion-focused PFA with someone using alcohol as self-medication may involve letting them vent about their problems. But Daria should make sure this does not escalate agitation. If it does, she should change the topic.

Stress Management–Focused

- If Megan seems sober enough to engage meaningfully, Daria can initiate a discussion of alternative ways to help her cope with the stress of her recent breakup.

Make a Plan

1. The immediate plan is getting Megan home, as described above.

2. The second plan is following up. Daria should make a point to check in later with Megan.

3. Once Megan is no longer intoxicated, Daria can offer hope by discussing ways she might begin to move on emotionally from her unexpected breakup.

4. Daria can suggest the option of professional counseling and, if needed, assist her in making the first appointment.

E-PFA Dialogue (It Might Sound Like This)

DARIA: Megan, I'm here to help you.

MEGAN (SLURRING HER WORDS): That's good. And maybe while you're helping me, we should have a drink. *(Raises her arm toward the server and becomes loud.)* I can't believe he did this.

DARIA (CALMLY): While I appreciate the offer of a drink, no thanks. And it seems that you don't need a drink either. It sounds like there's a lot you need to talk about, but I don't think this loud, crowded, environment is the best place to have that conversation.

MEGAN: You don't?

DARIA: No, I can barely hear you. And I want to make sure I'm hearing everything. Let me get you home, so we can talk.

MEGAN: I'm really drunk!

DARIA (CALMLY): I can see that. Have you taken anything else besides alcohol?

MEGAN: No. The alcohol is more than enough. At least for now.

DARIA: You don't need any other substances that could interact with the alcohol—and like I said, you also don't need any more alcohol.

MEGAN (REACHING INSIDE HER PURSE): Give me a few minutes to sober up and then if you want you can follow me home. (*Pulls out her keys.*)

DARIA: Considering how much you've been drinking in this short bit of time, you're going to need a lot more than a couple of minutes to sober up. Your blood alcohol level will go up before it starts going down, and you're in no condition to drive. So please give me your keys, and I will take care of your car and getting you home.

MEGAN: Then I should have another drink! That's the only way for me to deal with what he did!

DARIA: I'm sorry to hear about what your fiancé did. That's unthinkable, and I do want to hear more about it. But you've had so much to drink in such a short period of time, that's what we need to focus on first.

MEGAN: So, no more drinking?

DARIA (CALMLY): No, no more drinking. We need to get you home.

MEGAN: It's loud in here.

DARIA: I'm parked right outside. Let's walk to my car and I'll drive you home and stay with you. Have you paid your bar tab?

MEGAN: It's on my card.

DARIA (TO THE SERVER): My friend would like to close out her tab, please. (*The server returns with the bill and card. Daria adds the tip, shows Megan where to sign, then briefly speaks with the server, who nods to Daria.*)

MEGAN: What was that about?

DARIA: I asked if you could leave your car here overnight, and they said it was okay. We're going to walk to my car now—one step at a time together. I've got your purse, and I'm going to hold you around your waist like we're connected at the hip. Ready?

MEGAN (STAGGERING A BIT): Okay, if you say so. Let's do this!

(Daria helps Megan to the car, drives her home, and walks with her into the apartment, where Megan lives alone.)

MEGAN: I appreciate you getting me home, Daria. What about my car?

DARIA: I'm staying here tonight, and we'll go get it tomorrow morning.

MEGAN (SITTING ON THE COUCH): Okay, that's good.

DARIA: I like how you're sitting up, Megan. Keep doing that if you can. What else do you need?

MEGAN: Maybe I should have some coffee or take a cold shower to sober me up?

DARIA: Not a great idea. I know you are probably thirsty— alcohol will do that—but you should not eat or drink anything because you could choke or vomit it up later. The only thing that's going to sober you up is the passage of time.

MEGAN (BECOMING TEARFUL): Like the time I wasted for the past two years on someone who is nothing more than a liar and a cheat! How could I have been so wrong and foolish? You met him . . . did you see it?

DARIA: It's really awful that he did this to you. It sounds like it came completely out of nowhere. And for what it's worth, the several times I met him, I would have never guessed. He must be really good . . . at being really bad!

MEGAN (RAISING HER VOICE, TRYING TO STAND UP BUT FALLING BACK INTO A SEATED POSITION): I'm so furious about this. And I'm so embarrassed.

DARIA: You have every right to be upset about this. And there'll be plenty of time tomorrow to talk about ways to move on. But for now, do you want to sleep on the couch, or how about I walk you to your bed?

MEGAN: I need my bed. I just hope it isn't spinning.

DARIA: It might feel like it is from the alcohol, but sleeping on your side might help. Let me help you get you to your room.

MEGAN: Thanks, Daria.

DARIA: I'll sleep on the couch and will be here when you wake up tomorrow morning. We'll talk much more then.

MEGAN: Do you think I'm an alcoholic? Do I need help?

DARIA: We can talk about that tomorrow too, Megan. But know that I'll help you anyway you need.

Note: Daria should keep an eye on Megan. If Megan passes out and is breathing fewer than eight times per minute (slow breathing), if there are 10 seconds or more between breaths (irregular breathing), if her skin becomes clammy or blue-tinged and cold, if she begins vomiting while passed out and does not wake up, then this is a medical emergency. Daria should immediately call 9-1-1 and roll Megan onto her side to prevent choking (National Institute on Alcohol Abuse and Alcoholism [NIAAA], 2023).

ALCOHOL

SPECIFIC INTOXICANTS

The scenario with Megan and Daria involves a hypothetical case of alcohol intoxication. E-PFA is designed to be broadly applicable, regardless of the nature of the intoxicating substance. But effective crisis intervention relies on some knowledge of the substance(s) the person consumed.

Many substances besides alcohol alter consciousness and can lead to intoxication, even uncontrollable and potentially life-threatening intoxication. The rest of the chapter briefly reviews some of these substances. Still, when dealing with a highly intoxicated person, regardless of what has been consumed, it is best to err on the side of safety: Call for emergency medical assistance when in doubt about the person's well-being. Even consider calling for law enforcement assistance if the person is at risk of harming themselves or anyone else.

Alcohol

It is not surprising that most people associate intoxication with alcohol, as it's considered the oldest and most widely used psychoactive substance (Mirijello et al., 2023). For many, drinking alcohol is associated with enhancing a good time and is an integral part of celebrations, sporting events, and relaxed social occasions. However, drinking too much or drinking too quickly can lead to physical, behavioral, and emotional difficulties, including acute alcohol intoxication or, worse, alcohol overdose, which can be fatal. In a global study, alcohol use was the leading risk factor for disability among people aged 25 to 49 years (GBD 2019 Risk Factor Collaborators, 2020). According to the World Health Organization (2022), harmful alcohol use is responsible for three million deaths every year—5.3% of all deaths.

Before reviewing the specific signs and symptoms of mild to severe alcohol intoxication, it is helpful to provide perspective, as alluded to above, on what constitutes a standard alcoholic drink (or one alcoholic unit). In the United States, one standard drink is defined as containing 0.6 fluid ounces (14 grams) of ethanol. This translates to the following single servings (NIAAA, n.d.):

- 12 fluid ounces of beer at about 5% alcohol
- 5 fluid ounces of wine at about 12% alcohol
- 8–10 fluid ounces of malt liquor or flavored malt (e.g., hard seltzer) at about 7% alcohol
- 1.5 fluid ounces of distilled spirits (e.g., vodka, rum, tequila, whiskey) at 40% alcohol

Not surprisingly, what constitutes a standard drink varies by country.

The chemical compound ethanol is responsible for the intoxicating effects of alcoholic drinks. The ethanol passes through the digestive system into the bloodstream via the stomach and intestines. This results in a blood alcohol concentration (BAC) level, or blood alcohol level, which is the percentage of alcohol in one's bloodstream.

A blood test is the best way to determine BAC, but other methods, such as breath analysis, urine tests, and saliva tests, can be used. The central nervous system, which consists of the brain and spinal cord, is the primary site where ethanol exerts its effects. Once there, ethanol increases inhibition and decreases excitation, leading to many of the typical effects of intoxication. Naturally, the higher the BAC, the greater the percentage of ethanol in the bloodstream, resulting in more significant intoxication and impairment.

To provide context, a BAC of 0.08% is the legal limit to operate a vehicle in every US state but Utah (where it's 0.05%). As alluded to above, the number of drinks required to reach this limit depends on many factors. For example, individuals with lower body weight may reach this level after two drinks, while heavier people might need four drinks. There is considerable individual variability in the number of drinks needed to achieve a given BAC.

Another factor affecting BAC is how rapidly the drinks are consumed. Binge drinking, which is defined differently by various sources based on quantity (e.g., 4–6 drinks for women, 5–7 drinks for men), time frame (e.g., 2–3 hours), BAC levels (e.g., at least 0.08%), and frequency (e.g., 5–12 episodes in the past six months) is thought to occur in 17% of US adults and 29.5% of young adults (ages 18 to 25 years) (Centers for Disease Control and Prevention [CDC], 2024a; NIAAA, 2024). This results in an astonishing estimate of 17.5 billion total binge drinks annually in the United States in 2015; furthermore, and dishearteningly, more than half of the 88,000 US deaths from excessive drinking each year are attributed to binge drinking (Kanny et al., 2018).

Alcohol — Levels of Impairment

The following, adapted from NIAAA (2024) and other sources (Mirijello et al., 2023), outlines the clear signs of impairment, ranging from mild to life threatening, that may occur at various BAC levels.

MILD IMPAIRMENT (BAC 0.00–0.05%)

Signs of intoxication at this level include feelings or behaviors of:

- Relaxation
- Lightheadedness
- Slight impairment in balance and coordination
- Mild impairment in attention and speech
- Some social disinhibition

It has been suggested that BAC levels above 0.055% lead to "the point of diminishing returns" (McDonald, 2024).

MODERATE IMPAIRMENT (BAC 0.06–0.15%)

Signs of intoxication at this level include feeling or experiencing:

- A heightened buzz, which can range from increased euphoria or relaxation effects to feeling drunk
- More pronounced impairments in speech (e.g., talking louder) and attention
- Glassy-eyed appearance
- Greater issues with balance and coordination
- Mood changes, including signs of aggression
- Impairment in reaction time and skills needed for driving (recall that a 0.08% BAC is considered legally impaired)

SEVERE IMPAIRMENT (BAC 0.16 — 0.30%)

Signs of intoxication at this level include feelings or behaviors of:

- Increasing drunkenness
- Significant to gross disorientation
- Nausea
- Slurred speech
- Motor impairment
- Memory issues (feeling dazed)
- Impairment of driving-related skills
- Need for assistance with standing and walking
- Dangerously impaired judgment
- Stupor, potentially involving blackouts, vomiting, and loss of consciousness

LIFE-THREATENING IMPAIRMENT
(BAC 0.31–0.45%)

Signs of intoxication at this level include:

- Loss of consciousness
- Onset of coma
- Increased risk of death due to respiratory depression and cardiac arrest

Cannabis (Marijuana)

Cannabis sativa is a plant that contains about 540 substances, collectively referred to as cannabis. Of these, about 120 are cannabinoids, two of which are particularly relevant. One, cannabidiol (CBD), is nonintoxicating, and its derivatives have been reported by users to help in varying degrees with psychiatric conditions such as anxiety (see Chapter Eight), depression (see Chapter Five), autism spectrum symptoms, sleep, arthritis, multiple sclerosis, chronic pain, migraines, appetite loss, and nausea and vomiting associated with cancer treatments (Leas et al., 2020; Palrasu et al., 2022).

The other compound, delta-9 tetrahydrocannabinol (THC), is the main psychoactive compound in cannabis. It interacts with and disrupts certain brain and nervous system receptors, such as the receptor site for dopamine (which is involved in pleasure, reward, and motivation), and is responsible for the intoxicating sensation of being "high." Marijuana refers to cannabis that contains substantial amounts of THC.

The following are some of the ways THC can be ingested (Murphy et al., 2015; National Institute on Drug Abuse [NIDA], 2019):

- Cigarette form (rolled joints)
- Hollowed-out cigars (blunts)

- Dabbing—either smoking or vaping concentrates, often with a vape pen
- Glass pipes
- Bongs
- Edibles (e.g., gummies, brownies, hard candies)
- Beverages

Cannabis—Signs of Impairment

THC intoxication develops within minutes if cannabis is smoked, but may take several hours if ingested orally, with effects usually lasting up to four hours (CDC, 2024c).

The effects of THC intoxication include:

- Giddiness
- Relaxation
- Contentment
- Altered perceptions of time and space
- Enhanced sensory experiences
- Increased appetite (aka the munchies)
- Sleepiness
- Dry mouth

There is a dose-response relation with THC, with higher doses leading to more profound effects. Research has shown that long-term cannabis use (for several years or more) and heavy use (for most in the study, four or more days per week) are associated with cognitive decline, memory and attention problems, and smaller volume of the hippocampus (the part of the brain involved in memory) in midlife (Meier et al., 2022). Long-term cannabis use, particularly for those who smoked it, has been linked to several cardiovascular effects, including an increased risk of high blood pressure immediately after its use, stroke, and heart disease (CDC, 2024b).

Cannabis is cultivated in 154 countries, with an estimated 228 million users worldwide (United Nations Office on Drugs and Crime, 2024). According to the *DSM-5-TR* (American Psychiatric Association, 2022), the risk of acute toxicity of cannabinoids is low, but in rare instances such toxicity can be severe.

Cannabis was outlawed for any use (including medical purposes) when the Controlled Substances Act was passed in the United States in 1970. In 1996, California launched the first medical marijuana program, even though it conflicted with federal policy. In 2012 Colorado and Washington became the first two US states to legalize marijuana for recreational use. As of 2024, 24 states (plus DC) have fully legalized recreational marijuana use. In the first quarter of 2024, these states generated a combined total of more than $20 billion in tax revenue from legal sales (Marijuana Policy Project, n.d.). It is worth noting that current legal cannabis products often have higher THC potency than those from several decades ago (Smart et al., 2017).

In 2014, Uruguay became the first country in the world to legalize cannabis use nationwide, followed by Canada in 2018. A recent Canadian study showed that while there has been no overall increase in emergency visits for acute cannabis intoxication since legalization, there has been a 56% increase in reported use among young adults aged 18–29 years (Hall et al., 2023). As noted above, while cannabis use has become more widespread and socially accepted—especially with these recent legalization efforts—there seems to be growing and reasonably legitimate concerns about its long-term effects.

Cocaine

Cocaine is an addictive stimulant derived from the leaves of the coca plant, which is native to South America (Brain & Coward, 1989). The drug binds to the receptors for several neurochemicals and blocks their reuptake, creating an excess of these substances, including serotonin and norepinephrine, but most notably dopamine. Dopamine is responsible for motivation, reward, and pleasure, and its excess results in cocaine's characteristic "rush" of euphoric effects (Bravo et al., 2022; Richards & Le, 2023).

Cocaine has a powerful concurrent psychological addictiveness, leading users to seek and consume more. It is typically used in a powdered form and is most often ingested by snorting, with effects usually occurring within 1–3 minutes of ingestion and lasting for about 15–30 minutes (NIDA, 2016). Cocaine can also be processed into a solid crystal form, known as crack (due to the sound it makes when the crystal rocks are heated), which can be smoked. The effects of smoking crack cocaine are almost immediate, are typically more intense than snorting, and last a shorter time, about 5–15 minutes (NIDA, 2016).

Cocaine—Signs of Impairment

The signs and symptoms of moderately acute cocaine intoxication include:

- Dilated pupils
- Rapid speech
- Altered mental state
- Increased sex drive
- Restlessness
- Hypertension (elevated blood pressure)
- Impulsiveness
- Twitching
- Accelerated heart rate
- Sweating
- Chills
- Bloodshot eyes

- Difficulty getting to sleep
- Increased energy
- More confidence
- Anxiety and extreme paranoia
- Mood swings
- Repetitive sniffling
- Saddened mood (when effects wear off)

Cocaine—Signs of Overdose

Because the intoxicating effects of cocaine use can suddenly progress to an overdose—defined by the CDC (2024d) as an injury to the body from poisoning that jeopardizes health and safety when someone takes a drug in excessive amounts—it's important to be aware of the following signs and symptoms of a cocaine overdose (Bravo et al., 2022; NHSinform, 2023):

- Chest pain
- Stroke (mostly the result of increased blood pressure)
- Heart attack
- Respiratory failure
- Acute renal failure (with chronic use)
- Seizures
- Coma
- Abdominal pain
- Hyperthermia (high body temperature)
- Headache
- Liver damage

About 5 million Americans aged 12 years or older acknowledged using cocaine in 2023 (Substance Abuse and Mental Health Services Administration [SAMHSA], 2024), with worldwide estimates around 23 million (United Nations Office on Drugs and Crime, 2024). In 2021, more than 24,000 Americans died from an overdose involving cocaine, accounting for nearly 23% of all overdose deaths that year (Spencer et al., 2024). Death rates from cocaine use vary across countries, and no single global statistic exists for deaths attributed to cocaine or crack cocaine use.

Opioids

Opioids are medications designed to help manage severe pain and are intended for short-term use, such as after surgery. Between 1999 and 2010, the use of prescription opioids in the United States quadrupled (Guy et al., 2017). This massive increase was driven by several factors, including misleading marketing (e.g., claims that opioids were safe and nonaddictive for long-term use), unregulated distribution, and the proliferation of "pill mills" (medical practices that inappropriately prescribe large quantities of opioids without sufficient medical justification)—all of which contributed to the opioid epidemic in this country (Szalavitz, 2021). For example, out-of-state drug companies shipped nearly nine million pills to a coal mining town with fewer than 400 residents in West Virginia over two years (Eyre, 2020). To provide additional alarming context, in 2018, the United States had 5% of the world's population but consumed 80% of the world's opioids (American Council on Science and Health, 2018).

From 1999 to 2021, close to 645,000 people in the United States died from an overdose involving either prescription or illegal opioids (CDC, 2024e). Additionally, the number of people who died from a drug overdose in 2021 was more than six times higher than in 1999, and over 75% of drug overdose deaths in 2022 involved opioid use (CDC, 2024e).

Opioids work by affecting receptors in the brain to produce pain relief. The terms "opioid" and "opiate" are often used interchangeably, but there are differences between the two. Opiates are naturally occurring substances derived from the milky, latex sap of the opium poppy plant. In addition to opium, the most common opiates are morphine—isolated in 1803 as the active narcotic ingredient in opium (and about ten times more potent and incredibly addictive)—and codeine (Boysen et al., 2023).

Opioids are natural or synthetic substances that bind to opioid receptors in the brain, producing effects similar to those of opiates. They include (Kerrigan & Goldberger, 2020):

- *Heroin*—Derived from morphine (also known as diamorphine) and originally touted as a safer, less addictive alternative to morphine. As is now well known, heroin is fast acting and highly addictive. Heroin is one of the most pervasive illicit drugs, and when produced in underground laboratories, it is often laced with other chemicals (e.g., baking soda, talc, flour).
- *Methadone*—Most often used to reduce withdrawal symptoms in people addicted to other drugs (such as heroin) because it is effective when delivered orally and has moderately long-lasting effects.
- *Oxycodone*—The active ingredient in OxyContin (the brand name of a long-acting formulation) and Percocet (the brand name of a combination of oxycodone and acetaminophen).
- *Hydrocodone*—Similar to oxycodone but about 50% less potent. It stays in the system longer, and is often used for longer-lasting pain and in cough syrups.
- *Tramadol*—Commonly prescribed for round-the-clock management of moderate to severe pain. It has potency similar to codeine but has a lower risk of respiratory depression.
- *Fentanyl*—Has analgesic effects similar to morphine, but estimated to be up to 100 times stronger. It comes in a variety of forms, including nasal spray, transdermal patch, injection, and tablet. There are two types of fentanyl, pharmaceutical and illegally manufactured. Sadly, illicit fentanyl use has become more

widespread than its intended medical use. Just two milligrams of fentanyl can be lethal, and illicit producers frequently mix or substitute fentanyl with other street drugs to increase addition and profit (National Center for Drug Abuse Statistics, n.d.). In 2022 the United States Drug Enforcement Administration (DEA) seized more than 50 million pills laced with fentanyl, 60% of which contained a potentially lethal dose (DEA, 2022).

Opioids — Signs of Impairment

- Initial euphoria
- Absence of pain
- Slow pulse
- Confusion
- Delirium
- Constricted pupils
- Low body temperature
- Slurred speech
- Sedation
- Nausea and vomiting

Opiods — Signs of Overdose

Because opioid intoxication can quickly lead to an overdose, it's important to be aware of some of the common symptoms:

- Loss of consciousness
- Failure to respond to stimuli
- Gurgling noises
- Slowed or stopped breathing
- Clammy skin

Any suspected sign of an opioid overdose requires immediate medical attention (i.e., calling 9-1-1). In addition, naloxone is an over-the-counter medication approved by the US Food and Drug

Administration (FDA) that can reverse an opioid overdose (NIDA, 2022). It functions as an opioid antagonist, meaning it binds to the same receptors in the brain as the opioid (e.g., fentanyl, oxycodone, heroin, morphine). By attaching to these receptors, naloxone blocks and reverses the opioid's effects, including the slowing or stopping of breathing. Naloxone activates the respiratory centers, allowing the person to breathe again. It works in the body for up to 90 minutes, and can be administered as a prepackaged nasal spray or via injection. While not a treatment for opioid use disorder, naloxone can rapidly reverse an opioid overdose, prevent brain damage, and save a life.

MDMA (Ecstasy)

MDMA, or 3,4-methylenedioxymethamphetamine (now you know why it's called MDMA), is a synthetic drug with dual properties as both a stimulant and a hallucinogen. It is illegal in the United States, but its legal status varies in other countries. According to the National Institute on Drug Abuse (2017), it also has properties of an entactogen, which is a substance that increases self-awareness and empathy. MDMA is often referred to as ecstasy when used in tablet form, and as Molly (or Mandy) when used in a purer powder or capsule form. As with other drugs discussed in this chapter, the risk arises from substances marketed as ecstasy or Molly, as they may be laced or contaminated with other unknown, potentially harmful substances.

MDMA is most commonly associated with recreational use, particularly at raves (dance parties) and music festivals. The effects of MDMA usually begin within 30–45 minutes after ingesting one to two tablets, peak 15–30 minutes later, and last for about 3–6 hours, or sometimes longer (DEA, 2020). According to the 2021 National Survey on Drug Use and Health, about 2.2 million

U.S. adults reported using MDMA in the past year (SAMHSA, 2021).

MDMA—Signs of Impairment

Multiple effects are associated with MDMA intoxication, including:

- Feeling energized
- Time distortion
- Heightened overall sensory experiences, but often with poor perception of motion (making driving a vehicle quite dangerous)
- Reduced inhibitions
- Euphoria
- Seeking closeness
- Enhanced empathy
- Increased sexuality (potentially risky)

MDMA—Signs of Overdose

Fortunately, fatal overdoses from the use of pure (i.e., untainted) MDMA alone are rare (Pilgrim et al., 2011). Symptoms of overdose include:

- Hypertension
- Faintness
- Panic
- Seizures
- Loss of consciousness
- Hyperthermia (abnormally high body temperature)
- Feelings of depersonalization
- Nausea
- Sweating

MDMA was accidentally discovered in 1912 by Merck Pharmaceuticals and was initially considered to have little practical clinical use (Hallifax, 2022). It was more formally studied in 1953, when the US Army Chemical Center funded secret animal testing of various psychotropic chemicals, including MDMA, for their potential as "mind-control" or "truth-serum" drugs (Hallifax, 2022; Holland, 2001).

In the late 1970s and early 1980s, MDMA was studied and used therapeutically with reported success by an estimated 4,000 therapists in California; however, this use was not publicized. Its clandestine status was likely a response to what had happened with lysergic acid diethylamide (LSD), which had been extensively studied and used therapeutically in the early to mid-1960s. LSD was banned in 1968, and in 1970 the US Congress passed the Controlled Substances Act, classifying LSD and other hallucinogens, such as psilocybin (see below) as Schedule I drugs—defined as extremely dangerous and without medical value (DEA, 2018). This classification was largely influenced by the widespread recreational use and adverse effects associated with these substances, particularly among members of the counterculture or "hippie" movement.

By the early 1980s, MDMA's underground recreational use, particularly as a party or "rave" drug, had expanded widely. This rise in use, along with mounting legislative pressure, led the DEA to classify MDMA as a Schedule I drug in 1985, placing it alongside LSD and psilocybin (Holland, 2001). This designation effectively halted clinical research on MDMA-assisted psychotherapy research in the United States. But other countries, such as Switzerland, continued to investigate its therapeutic potential through the late 1980s and into the 1990s. Tensions persisted between those who argued that MDMA could be safely used in controlled clinical settings and those who pushed for prohibition to curb

recreational use. Undeterred, researchers obtained special per-
missions, and more than two decades later, the first controlled
clinical study of MDMA-assisted psychotherapy was published in
2010 (Mithoefer et al., 2010).

MDMA affects many of the same brain neurochemicals as cocaine; however, it has a greater impact on norepinephrine and
serotonin—the latter of which plays a primary role in mood, cognition, and perception—than on dopamine. MDMA has also
been shown to elevate levels of oxytocin (known as the attraction
or "love" hormone) and to decrease activity in the amygdala, the
brain region involved in processing emotions, particularly fear
(Dumont et al., 2009; Gamma et al., 2000). Because of these neurochemical effects—and the resulting behavioral effects, such as
feeling less defensive, less fearful, and more open to experience
without memory suppression—there has been a renewed push in
the past decade to study MDMA in controlled settings in combination with psychotherapy. Specifically, MDMA-assisted therapy
has been used to treat trauma-related disorders (e.g., PTSD, see
Chapter Eleven), especially among individuals who are resistant
to conventional treatments and struggle to form trusting relationships or to talk about topics they have avoided (Morgan, 2020).

Although MDMA is still classified as an illegal substance, the
FDA designated it as a "breakthrough therapy" for the treatment
of PTSD in 2017. This seeming contradiction reflects both the
rapid progress in exploring MDMA's therapeutic potential and the
differing roles of regulatory agencies in the United States.

Psilocybin

The psychedelic, or mind-altering, properties of some plants and
fungi have been known and used by humans for thousands of
years for medicinal, religious, and recreational purposes (Sharma
et al., 2023). Fungi, primarily mushrooms, are the principal

sources of these substances. Psilocybin is a hallucinogenic extract contained in certain types of mushrooms that grow on nearly every continent but are mostly found in the United States, Mexico, and Central America (Meyer & Slot, 2023). Known as "magic mushrooms," "sacred mushrooms," or "shrooms," they are usually brown or tan in color and are consumed orally—either raw, boiled in water to make tea, or cooked into foods—in fresh or dried forms. The dried form contains about 10 times more psilocybin. Not surprisingly, individual responses to psilocybin vary, but when it is taken orally, its hallucinogenic effects typically occur in 10–40 minutes and peak in 60–90 minutes (Lowe et al., 2021).

How psilocybin works is not yet completely understood. It is known that the body metabolizes psilocybin into psilocin, its main psychoactive component, which increases serotonin levels in the front part of the brain—the prefrontal cortex (NIDA, 2024). As noted earlier, serotonin is involved in mood, cognition, and perception. This increase appears to change activity in the anterior cingulate cortex, also located in the prefrontal cortex, resulting in temporary dysregulation or "disintegration" of brain activity and connectivity. For example, some brain waves slow, but others speed up, affecting self-awareness, emotional regulation, and thinking. These effects, when combined with others, seem to allow the brain to rely less on prior beliefs, making it more open to new information. Over time, this may contribute to a broadening of brain network integration (Daws et al., 2022; Golden & Chadderton, 2022).

Psilocybin—Signs of Impairment

Some of the behavioral and physiological signs and symptoms of psilocybin intoxication include:

- Mild relaxation
- Giddiness

- Visual enhancement (e.g., seeing colors brighter)
- Visual disturbances (e.g., seeing things moving)
- Sensory distortions that may be accompanied by feelings of anxiety or impaired judgment of time
- Spiritual awakening
- Lack of coordination
- Dizziness
- Nausea
- Shivering
- Agitation
- Muscle weakness
- Mildly to moderately increased heart rate
- Increased breathing rate

Psilocybin has a low level of toxicity, meaning a low potential for fatal overdose, unlike the high levels noted for opioids and cocaine. There are, however, associated health risks, such as operating a vehicle while impaired, or experiencing panic or extreme fear, which under the influence could lead to dangerous behavioral decisions.

The results of a recent study showed the lifetime prevalence of psilocybin use among adults aged 18 years and older in the United States grew from about 25 million in 2019 to around 31 million in 2023 (Rockhill et al., 2025). Prior to 2019, psilocybin use was noted to be relatively stable. In 2023, its use increased 44% among those aged 18 to 29 years and 188% among those 30 years and older. While accurate worldwide prevalence is difficult to determine, a 2017 global survey found that about 20.6% of people who acknowledged using any drugs reported using mushrooms within their lifetime (Mikulic, 2021). Considering the date of this global survey, as well as the recently noted proliferation in the United States, it seems reasonable that the current global prevalence rates are higher.

Research into the possible therapeutic use of psilocybin began in the late 1950s, and during the 1960s Sandoz Pharmaceuticals distributed a pill containing two milligrams of psilocybin for studies on brain function, recidivism, and the enhancement of religious experiences among divinity students (Lowe, 2021). Nevertheless, as noted above, the late 1960s saw a dramatic increase in recreational drug use in the United States, prompting Congress and the DEA to prohibit substances like psilocybin, LSD, and mescaline (a psychedelic derived from the peyote cactus) in 1970.

In 2000, the Johns Hopkins University School of Medicine, under the direction of Dr. Roland Griffiths, obtained approval to conduct research with psychedelics in the United States. In 2006 he and his colleagues published a landmark study demonstrating the positive long-term effects of a single high dose of psilocybin (Griffiths et al., 2006). Since then, Johns Hopkins has published more than 150 research articles on the use of psilocybin to help treat major depression, addictions (e.g., smoking, alcohol), eating disorders, distress associated with life-threatening illnesses, and obsessive-compulsive disorder (Johns Hopkins Center for Psychedelic & Consciousness Research, n.d.).

In 2019, the FDA, as it had previously done with MDMA, designated psilocybin as a "breakthrough therapy" for the treatment of treatment-resistant depression and major depressive disorder, despite its current classification as a Schedule I drug.

Ketamine

Ketamine, developed in the early 1960s, was originally used as an anesthetic (a substance that suppresses responses to sensory stimulation) in human and veterinary medicine. Unlike traditional anesthetics, however, it induces a dreamlike, out-of-body state, leading to its classification as a "dissociative anesthetic" (Hirota & Lambert, 2022). Ketamine also has analgesic (pain-relieving) properties and is notable for producing its effects without adversely affecting one's breathing rate.

Unlike MDMA and psilocybin, ketamine was approved for human use by the FDA in 1970. It is currently classified as a Schedule III controlled substance under the Controlled Substance Act, meaning it is approved for medical use, has a low to moderate risk of abuse, and is subject to strict regulations regarding its manufacturing, distribution, and use (DEA, 2018; Mion, 2017). As with MDMA, ketamine's classification and legal status vary across countries.

Ketamine is typically administered intravenously (IV), intramuscularly, as a nasal spray, or in tablet, powder, pill, liquid, lozenge, or sublingual (under the tongue) form (National Pain Centers, 2021). Depending on how it's delivered and individual factors such as body size, its effects typically begin within minutes and last between 30 minutes and one hour, though IV administration can extend effects up to four hours (Rosenbaum et al., 2024).

Ketamine — Signs of Impairment

Signs and symptoms of recreational ketamine intoxication include:

- Euphoric rush
- Out-of-body experiences
- Sensation of dissolving into one's surroundings
- Laughter
- Tearfulness
- Salivation
- Detachment from reality
- Confusion
- Dizziness
- Jerky muscle movements

Ketamine—Signs of an Overdose

Although a ketamine overdose is uncommon, it can have serious complications, particularly if ketamine is used in conjunction with alcohol. Signs and symptoms of an overdose include:

- Inability to move
- Periods of stopped breathing
- Nausea
- Prolonged visual disturbances
- Seizures
- Cardiac arrest
- Short-term memory loss

In the late 1990s in London and the early 2000s in the United States, ketamine became an increasingly popular recreational "club drug," often snorted in its powdered form, leading to rapid effects. Due to its notable short-term memory loss effects (described in more detail below), ketamine has unfortunately been used as a date-rape drug (Albright et al., 2012).

According to data collected from 2015–2019 and published in 2023, an estimated 0.13% of adults (more males than females) in the United States had reportedly used ketamine for nonmedical purposes in the past year (Yockey, 2023). Despite this seemingly low reported prevalence rate, ketamine use has increased considerably over the past ten years, and ketamine-related poisonings in the United States have risen by 81% in the past several years (Palamar et al., 2021). From 2018 to 2022, 81 countries across all continents reported the illegal manufacturing and marketing of ketamine substances (United Nations Office on Drugs and Crime, 2022).

The potential for ketamine to be used in mental health treatment dates back to the 1970s and became more formalized in the 1990s. Over the past two decades, growing evidence has supported ketamine as an effective rapid-acting antidepressant for individuals with treatment-resistant depression. For example, ketamine infusions have been shown to deliver effects within two hours (compared to the weeks it typically takes other antidepressant medications) and to provide benefits lasting up to seven days (Zarate et al., 2006). In 2019, the accumulation of evidence led the FDA to approve the nasal spray esketamine (a ketamine derivative). The medication is meant to be administered and closely monitored in a provider's office as part of a comprehensive treatment plan that may include psychotherapy and oral antidepressants.

Ketamine's antidepressant effects are thought to result from its ability to enhance communication between neurons in the prefrontal cortex, which, as noted previously, is responsible for reasoning, planning, and abstract thinking, and the hippocampus, involved in memory. The dissociative effects of ketamine are thought to occur in the rear part of the brain — specifically, the posteromedial cortex (Powell, 2023). In addition, ketamine blocks the activity of NMDA receptors in the brain, an effect that boosts levels of the neurochemical glutamate. This increase in glutamate is thought to make the brain more adaptable and to foster the creation of new neural pathways, leading to more positive thoughts and behaviors (Powell, 2023). Researchers are now working to find the right balance between optimizing antidepressant effects and minimizing dissociative effects.

Ketamine has been shown to help with suicidal ideation (see Chapter Sixteen) and refractory epileptic seizures (those that do not respond to other medications). It has been investigated with varying degrees of success for posttraumatic stress disorder (see Chapter Eleven), obsessive-compulsive disorder, substance use disorder, and anorexia nervosa (see Chapter Twelve) (Abbar et al., 2022; Alkhachroum et al., 2020; Ragnhildstveit et al., 2022; Walsh et al., 2022).

A Word of Caution About the Combined
Effects of Intoxicants

These brief reviews aim to inform readers about the intoxicating and potentially overdose effects of individual substances, yet it is clear—and unfortunate—that many of them are often combined, particularly for recreational use. In combination, these substances can cause extreme depersonalization, profound sedation, respiratory distress, coma, and potentially fatal outcomes. The Centers for Disease Control and Prevention (2022) reports that nearly 50% of overdose deaths result from multiple drug use.

References

Abbar, M., Demattei, C., El-Hage, W., Llorca, P-M., Samalin, L., Demaricourt, P., Gaillard, R., Courtet, P., Vaiva, G., Gorwood, P., Fabbro, P., & Jollant, F. (2022). Ketamine for the acute treatment of severe suicidal ideation: Double blind, randomised placebo controlled trial. *BMJ, 376,* e067194. https://dx.doi.org/10.1136/bmj-2021-067194

Albright, J. A., Stevens, S. A., & Beussman, D. J. (2012). Detecting ketamine in beverage residues: Application in date rape detection. *Drug Testing and Analysis, 4*(5), 337–341. https://doi.org/10.1002/dta.335

Alkhachroum, A., Der-Nigoghossian, C. A., Matthews, E., Massad, N., Letchinger, R., Doyle, K., Chiu W.-T., Kromm, J., Rubinos, C., Velazquez, A., Roh, D., Agarwal, S., Park, S., Connolly, E. S., & Claassen, J. (2020). Ketamine to treat super-refractory status epilepticus. *Neurology, 95*(16), e2286–e2294. https://dx.doi.org/10.1212/WNL.0000000000010611

American Council on Science and Health. (2018). *Opioid epidemic's global spread, explained.* https://www.acsh.org/news/2018/08/21/opioid-epidemics-global-spread-explained-13330

American Psychiatric Association. (2022). Substance-related and addictive disorders. In *Diagnostic and statistical manual of mental disorders* (5th ed., text rev.). https://doi.org/10.1176/appi.books.9780890425787.x16_Substance_Related_Disorders

Boysen, P. G., Patel, J. H., & King, A. N. (2023). Brief history of opioids in perioperative and periprocedural medicine to inform the future. *Ochsner Journal, 23*(1), 43–49. https://doi.org/10.31486/toj.22.0065

Brain, P. F., & Coward, G. A. (1989). A review of the history, actions, and legitimate uses of cocaine. *Journal of Substance Abuse, 1*(4), 431–451. https://doi.org/10.1016/S0899-3289(20)30007-9

Bravo, R. R., Faria, A. C., Brito-da-Costa, A. M., Carmo, H., Mladěnka, P., da Silva, D. D., Remião, F., on behalf of the OEMONOM Researchers. (2022). Cocaine: An updated overview on chemistry, detection, biokinetics, and pharmacotoxicological aspects including abuse pattern. *Toxins, 14*, 278. https://doi.org/10.3390/toxins14040278

Centers for Disease Control and Prevention. (2022). *Polysubstance use facts.* https://www.cdc.gov/stopoverdose/polysubstance-use/index.html

Centers for Disease Control and Prevention. (2024a). *Alcohol and public health data on excessive drinking.* https://www.cdc.gov/alcohol/data-stats.htm

Centers for Disease Control and Prevention. (2024b). *Cannabis and heart health.* https://www.cdc.gov/cannabis/health-effects/heart-health.html

Centers for Disease Control and Prevention. (2024c). *Cannabis and public health.* https://www.cdc.gov/cannabis/health-effects/poisoning.html

Centers for Disease Control and Prevention. (2024d). *Overdose prevention: Commonly used terms.* https://www.cdc.gov/overdoes-prevention/glossary

Centers for Disease Control and Prevention. (2024e). *Overdose prevention: Understanding the opioid overdose epidemic.* https://www.cdc.gov/oversoes-prevention/about/understanding-the-opioid-overdose-epidemic.html

Daws, R. E., Timmermann, C., Giribaldi, B., Sexton, J. D., Wall, M. B., Erritzoe, D., Roseman, L., Nutt, D., & Carhart-Harris, R. (2022). Increased global integration in the brain after psilocybin therapy for depression. *Nature Medicine, 28*, 844–851. https://doi.org/10.1038/s41591-022-01744-z

Dumont, G. J. H., Sweep, F. C. G. J., van der Steen, R., Hermsen, R., Donders, A. R. T., Touw, D. J., van Gerven, J. M. A., Buitelaar, J. K., & Verkes, R. J. (2009). Increased oxytocin concentrations and prosocial feelings in humans after ecstasy (3,4-methylenedioxymethamphetami ne) administration. *Social Neuroscience, 4*(4), 359–366. https://doi.org /10.1080/17470910802649470

Eyre, E. (2020). *Death in Mud Lick: A coal country fight against the drug companies that delivered the opioid epidemic.* Simon and Schuster.

Gamma, A., Buck, A., Berthold, T., Hell, D., & Vollenweider, F. X. (2000). 3,4-methylenedioxymethamphetamine (MDMA) modulates cortical and limbic brain activity as measured by [$H_2^{15}O$]-PET in healthy humans. *Neuropsychopharmacology, 23*(4), 388–395. https:// doi.org/10.1016/S0893-133X(00)00130-5

GBD 2019 Risk Factor Collaborators. (2020). Global burden of 87 risk factors in 204 countries and territories, 1990–2019: A systematic analysis for the Global Burden of Disease Study 2019. *Lancet, 396,* 1223–1249. https://doi.org/10.1016/s0140-6736(20)30752-2

Golden, C. T., & Chadderton, P. (2022). Psilocybin reduces low frequency oscillatory power and neuronal phase-locking in the anterior cingulate cortex of awake rodents. *Scientific Reports, 12,* 12702. https://doi.org/10.1038/s41598-022-16325-w

Griffiths, R. R., Richards, W. A., McCann, U., & Jesse, R. (2006). Psilocy- bin can occasion mystical-type experiences having substantial and sustained personal meaning and spiritual significance. *Psychopharma- cology, 187*(3), 268–283. https://doi.org/10.1007/s00213-006-0475-5

Guy, G. P., Zhang, K., Bohm, M. K., Losby, J., Lewis, B., Young, R., Murphy, L. B., & Dowell, D. (2017). Vital signs: Changes in opioid prescribing in the United States, 2006–2015. *Morbidity and Mortality Weekly Report, 66*(26), 697–704. https://doi.org/10.15585/mmwr.mm6626a4

Hall, W., Stjepanović, D., Dawson, D., & Leung, J. (2023). The implemen- tation and public health impacts of cannabis legalization in Canada: A systematic review. *Addiction, 118*(11), 2062–2072. https://doi.org/10.1111 /add.16274

Hallifax, J. (2022, May). A brief history of MDMA: From CIA to raves to psychedelic therapy. *Psychedelic Spotlight.* https:// psychedelicspotlight.com/history-of-mdma-cia-raves-psychedelic therapy/

Hirota, K., & Lambert, D. G. (2022). Ketamine: History and role in anesthetic pharmacology. *Neuropharmacology, 216.* https://doi.org/10 .1016/j.neuropharm.2022.109171

Holland, J. (2001). The history of MDMA. In J. Holland (Ed.), *Ecstasy: The complete guide: A comprehensive look at the risks and benefits of MDMA* (pp. 11–20). Park Street Press.

Johns Hopkins Center for Psychedelic & Consciousness Research. (n.d.). https://hopkinspsychedelic.org/about

Kanny, D., Naimi, T. S., Liu, Y., Lu, H., & Brewer, R. D. (2018). Annual total binge drinks consumed by U.S. adults, 2015. *American Journal of Preventive Medicine, 54*(4), 486–496. https://doi.org/10.1016/j.amepre.2017.12.021

Kerrigan, S., & Goldberger, B. A. (2020). Opioids. In B. S. Levine & S. Kerrigan (Eds.), *Principles of forensic toxicology* (pp. 347–369). Springer.

Leas, E. C., Hendrickson, E. M., Nobles, A. L., Todd, R., Smith, D. M., Dredze, M., & Ayers, J. W. (2020). Self-reported cannabidiol (CBD) use for conditions with proven therapies. *JAMA Network/Open, 3*(10), e2020977. https://doi.org/jamanetworkopen.2020.20977

Lowe, H., Toyang, N., Steele, B., Valentine, H., Grant, J., Ali, A., Ngwa, W., & Gordon, L. (2021). The therapeutic potential of psilocybin. *Molecules, 26*(10). https://doi.org/10.3390/molecules26102948

Marijuana Policy Project. (n.d.). *Cannabis tax revenue in states that regulate cannabis for adult use.* https://www.mpp.org/issues/legalization/cannabis-tax-revenue-states-regulate-cannabis-adult-use

McDonald, J. E. (2024). *What is intoxication?* Center for student well-being. University of Notre Dame, Office of Student Affairs.

Meier, M. H., Caspi, A., Knodt, A. R., Hall, W., Ambler, A., Harrington, H., Hoban, S., Houts, R. M., Poulton, R., Ramrakha, S., Hariri, A. R., Moffitt, T. E. (2022). Long-term cannabis use and cognitive reserves and hippocampal volume in midlife. *The American Journal of Psychiatry, 179*(5). https://doi.org/10.1176/appi.ajp.2021.21060664

Merriam-Webster. (n.d.). *Definition of "intoxication."* https://www.merriam-webster.com/dictionary/intoxication

Meyer, M., & Slot, J. (2023). The evolution and ecology of psilocybin in nature. *Fungal Genetics and Biology, 167.* https://doi.org/10.1016/j.fgh.2023.103812

Mikulic, M. (2021, March). *Global lifetime drug use of select types of drugs as of 2017.* Statista. https://www.statista.com/statistics/748239/global-lifetime-use-of-select-types-of-drugs/

Mion, G. (2017). History of anaesthesia: The ketamine story—past, present and future. *European Journal of Anaesthesiology, 34*(9), 571–575. https://doi.org/10.1097/EJA0000000000000638

Mirijello, A., Sestito, L., Antonelli, M., Gasbarrini, A., & Addolorate, G. (2023). Identification and management of acute alcohol intoxication.

European Journal of Internal Medicine, 108, 1–8. https://doi.org/10.1016/j
.ejim.2022.08.013

Mithoefer, M. C., Wagner, M. T., Mithoefer, A. T., Jerome, L., & Doblin,
R. (2010). The safety and efficacy of +3,4-methylenedioxymethamph
etaimine-assisted psychotherapy in subjects with chronic, treatment-
resistant posttraumatic stress disorder: The first randomized
controlled pilot study. *Journal of Psychopharmacology, 25*(4). https://
doi.org/10.1177/0269881110378371

Morgan, L. (2020). MDMA-assisted psychotherapy for people diagnosed with treatment-resistant PTSD: What it is and what it isn't.
Annals of General Psychiatry, 19, 33. https://doi.org/10.1186/s12991-020
-00283-6

Murphy, F., Sales, P., Murphy, S., Averill, S., Lau, N., & Sye-Ok, S.
(2015). Baby boomers and cannabis delivery systems. *Journal of Drug
Issues, 45*(3). https://doi.org/10.1177/0022042615580991

National Center for Drug Abuse Statistics. (n.d.). *Fentanyl abuse
statistics.* https://drugabusestatistics.org/fentanyl-abuse-statistics/

National Institute on Alcohol Abuse and Alcoholism. (n.d.). *Patient
education: What is a "standard" drink?* https://www.niaaa.nih.gov
/default/files/patient-education-drink-sizes-and-drinking-levels
.pdf

National Institute on Alcohol Abuse and Alcoholism. (2023). *Understanding the dangers of alcohol overdose.* https://www.niaaa.nih.gov
/publications/brochures-and-fact-sheets/understanding -dangers
-of-alcohol-overdose

National Institute on Alcohol Abuse and Alcoholism. (2024). *Understanding binge drinking.* https://www.niaaa.nih.gov/sites/default/files
/publicatications/NIAAA-Binge-Drinking-3.pdf

National Institute on Drug Abuse. (2016). *Cocaine.* https://nida.nih.gov
/sites/default/files/1141-cocaine.pdf

National Institute on Drug Abuse. (2017). *MDMA (Ecstasy) abuse
research report: What is MDMA?* https://nida.nih.gov/publications
/research-reports/mdma-ecstasy-abuse/what-mdma

National Institute on Drug Abuse. (2019). *Cannabis (marijuana) drug
facts.* https://nida.hih.gov/publications/drugfacts/cannabis-mari-
juana

National Institute on Drug Abuse. (2022). *Naloxone drug facts.* https://
nida.nih.gov/publications/drugfacts/naloxone

National Institute on Drug Abuse. (2024). *Psilocybin (magic mush-rooms)*. https://nida.nih.gov/research-topics/psilocybin-magic-mushrooms#is-psilocybin-safe

National Pain Centers. (2021). *Routes of administration*. https://www.nationalpain.com/routes-of-administration

NHSinform. (2023). *Cocaine*. https://www.nhsinform.scot/healthy-living/drugs-and-drug-use/common-drugs/cocaine

Palamar, J. J., Rutherford, C., & Keyes, K. M. (2021). Trends in ketamine use, exposures, and seizures in the United States up to 2019. *American Journal of Public Health, 111*(11), 2046–2049. https://doi.org/10.2105/AJPH.2021.306486

Palrasu, M., Wright, L., Patel, M., Leech, L., Branch, S., Harrelson, S., & Khan, S. (2022). Perspectives on challenges in cannabis drug delivery systems: Where are we? *Medical Cannabis and Cannabinoids, 5*(1), 102–119. https://doi.org/10.1159/00

Pilgrim, J. L., Gerostamoulos, D., & Drummer, O. H. (2011). Deaths involving MDMA and the concomitant use of pharmaceutical drugs. *Journal of Analytical Toxicology, 35*(4), 219–226. https://doi.org/10.1093/anatox/35.4.219

Powell, A. (2023). The brain on ketamine. *Harvard Gazette*. https://news.harvard.edu/gazette/story/2023/05/how-ketamine-affects-three-regions-of-brain

Ragnhildstveit, A., Slayton, M., Jackson, L. K., Brendle, M., Ahuja, S., Holle, W., Moore, C., Sollars, K., Seli, P., & Robison, R. (2022). Ketamine as a novel psychopharmacotherapy for eating disorders: Evidence and future directions. *Brain Science, 12*(3), 382. https//doi.org/10.3390/brainsci12030382

Richards, J. R., & Le, J. K. (2023). *Cocaine toxicity*. National Library of Medicine. https://www.ncbi.nlm.nih.gov/books/NBK430976

Rockhill, K. M., Black, J. C., Ladka, M. S., Sumbundu, K. B., Olsen, H. A., Jewell, J. S., Hunt, J., Wolf, C., Nerurkar, K., Dart, R. C., & Monte, A. A. (2025). The rise of psilocybin use in the United States: A multisource observational study. *Annals of Internal Medicine*. https://doi.org/10.7326/ANNALS-24-03145

Rosenbaum, S. B., Gupta, V., Patel, P., & Palacios, J. L. (2024. *Ketamine*. Europe PMC. https://europepmc.org/article/nbk/nbk470357

Sharma, P., Nguyen, A. A., Matthews, S. J., Carpenter, E., Mathews, D. B., Patten, C. A., & Hammond, C. J. (2023). Psilocybin history, action and reaction: A narrative clinical review. *Journal of Psycho-pharmacology, 37*(9). https://doi.org/10.1177/02698811231190858

Smart, R., Caulkins, J. P., Kilmer, B., Davenport, S., & Midgette, G. (2017). Variation in cannabis potency and prices in a newly legal market: Evidence from 30 million cannabis sales in Washington state. *Addiction, 112*(12), 2167–2177.

Spencer, M. R., Garnett, M. F., & Miniño, A. M. (2024). *Drug overdose deaths in the United States, 2002–2022,* NCHS Data Brief, no 491. National Center for Health Statistics. https://doi.org/10.15620/cdc .135849

Strumila, R., Nobile, B., Korsakova, L., Lengvenyte, A., Olie, E., Lopez-Castroman, J., Guillaume, S., & Courtet, P. (2021). Psilocybin, a naturally occurring indoleamine compound, could be useful to prevent suicidal behaviors. *Pharmaceuticals, 14*(12), 1213. https://doi .org/10.2290/ph14121213

Substance Abuse and Mental Health Services Administration. (2022). *2021 national survey on drug use and health (NSDUH).* https://www .samhsa.gov/data/release/2021-national-survey-drug-use-and -health-nsduh-releases

Substance Abuse and Mental Health Services Administration. (2024). *Key substance use and mental health indicators in the United States: Results from the 2023 National Survey on Drug Use and Health.* https:// www.samhsa.gov/data/report/2023-nsduh-annual-national-report

Szalavitz, M. (2021, May). We're overlooking a major culprit in the opioid crisis. *Scientific American.* https://www.scientificamerican .com/article/were-overlooking-a-major-culprit-in-the-opioid-crisis

United Nations Office on Drugs and Crime. (2022). *"Tuci," "happy water," "k-powdered milk": Is the illicit market for ketamine expanding?* https://www.unodc.org/documents/scientific/Global_SMART _Update_2022_Vol.27.pdf

United Nations Office on Drugs and Crime. (2024). UNODC *World Drug Report 2024:* https://www.unodc.org/unodc/en/data-and -analysis/world-drug-report-2024.html

United States Drug Enforcement Administration. 2018. *Drug schedul-ing.* https://www.dea.gov/drug-information/drug-scheduling

United States Drug Enforcement Administration. 2020. *Drug fact sheet: Ecstasy/MDMA.* https://www.dea.gov/sites/default/files/2020-06 /Ecstasy-MDMA-2020_0.pdf

United States Drug Enforcement Administration. (2022). *DEA laboratory testing reveals that 6 out of 10 fentanyl-laced fake prescription pills now contain a potentially lethal dose of fentanyl, 2022.* https://www .dea.gov/alert/dea-laboratory-testing-reveals-6-out-of-10-fentanyl -laced-fake-prescription-pills-now-contain

Walsh, Z., Mollaahmetoglu, O. M., Rootman, J., Golsof, S., Keeler, J., Marsh, B., Nutt, D. J., & Morgan, C. J. A. (2022). Ketamine for the treatment of mental health and substance use disorders: Comprehensive systematic review. *BJPsych Open, 8*(1), 1–12. https://doi.org /10.1192/bjo.2021.1061

World Health Organization. (2022). *Alcohol.* https://www.who.int/news -room/fact-sheets/detail/alcohol

Yockey, A., & King, K. (2021). Use of psilocybin ("mushrooms") among US adults: 2015–2018. *Journal of Psychedelic Studies, 5*(1), 17–21. https://doi.org/10.1556/2054.2020.00159

Yockey, R. A. (2023). Past-year ketamine use: Evidence from a United States population, 2015–2019. *Journal of Psychoactive Drugs, 55*(2), 134–140. https//doi.org/10.1080/02791072.2022.2058896

Zarate, C. A., Singh, J. B., Carlson, P. J., Brutsche, N. E., Ameli, R., Luckenbaugh, D. A., Carney, D. S., & Manji, H. K. (2006). A randomized trial of an N-methyl-D-aspartate antagonist in treatment-resistant major depression. *JAMA Psychiatry, 63*(8), 856–864. https://doi.org/10.1001/archpsyc.63.8.856

FOURTEEN | Guilt, Regret, Shame

ANDREW IS A 50-YEAR-OLD SUCCESSFUL ATTOR-
NEY *who got divorced from his wife of twenty years about
two years ago. When Andrew graduated from law school in
2000, he went directly into a successful practice that special-
ized in international law. The hours were long, and his work
involved a lot of international travel that took him away
from his home and family. Promotions came rapidly, as
did salary increases. Over time, however, his marriage
eroded, accelerated by an affair he had, which ultimately led
to his divorce when his two sons were 14 and 16 years of age.*

*Now, on the eve of his oldest son's high school gradua-
tion — a milestone moment — Andrew finds himself reflecting
on his life, especially his marriage and relationship with his
children. He has grown increasingly sad and lethargic. A colleague at work, Jasmine, has noticed his persistent low mood
and asks if he is okay. Andrew candidly replies, "No, I'm not.
To be honest, I'm consumed with guilt over how I neglected my
marriage and my family. I put my career ahead of my marriage, had an affair, and my wife divorced me. I put my career*

ahead of my children, and they hardly know me." Jasmine asks if An-
drew would like to talk about it over lunch the next day. He agrees.

What Is Guilt?

Guilt is a common but unpleasant human emotion that we've all
experienced to some degree. At its core, guilt is the belief that one
is responsible or at fault for a perceived offense or wrongdoing.
There are generally recognized to be four types of guilt:

1) Guilt for doing something you should not have
2) Guilt for not doing something you should have
3) Guilt by association
4) Survivor's guilt (often felt by accident survivors, survivors of
   violence, or military personnel)

Key Features: Signs and Symptoms

Guilt is unique in that it functions as both an emotion and a cognition (thought). It usually combines sadness with remorse in response to an action you believe has caused harm or violated your
moral principles. Though often less intense than other emotions,
guilt tends to linger and can be gnawing. While guilt can have a
negative impact on our lives, it can also be useful in regulating social behavior. It can motivate us to make amends for our actions
and avoid future wrongdoing. But when guilt becomes overwhelming or persistent enough to interfere with daily life, it
turns maladaptive.

Reasons People Feel Guilty

A national survey asked people why they felt guilty. The results
identified 1,515 reasons, which were classified into 12 content

categories. The most frequently reported reason was "Telling lies/withholding truth/information." The second most common was "Not spending (enough) time with family members/Not taking (enough) care of family members/Not being there for family members." Male and female participants had different reasons for feeling guilty. Women's feelings of guilt related to family members and children, and more specifically to failing to care for others. Men, by contrast, tended to cite guilt over "Misconduct/mistakes being made or because of difficulties in marriage/relationship" (Luck & Luck-Sikorski, 2022).

With the rise of social media, especially the increase in cyberbullying, guilt has, unfortunately, become weaponized. For example, about half of students between ages 13 and 17 years report having been cyberbullied (Cyberbullying Research Center, 2024).

Understanding Guilt, Regret, and Shame

Guilt often gives rise to regret. Regret involves accepting responsibility for a perceived offense or wrongdoing and feeling remorseful about it. It is often related to thoughts of contrition or repentance, and can lead to corrective actions — or even preventive ones — in the future. In this way, regret can be a natural, healthy response to guilt — unless, however, regret leads to shame.

Shame is the angst and distress associated with more extreme guilt. It involves feelings of humiliation and a loss of honor or respect. Shame can amplify the stress of regret. Shame is not healthy and serves no useful purpose. In fact, its harmful, if not toxic, effects are commonly associated with cyberbullying. Shame is closely tied to feelings of inferiority and worthlessness rooted in the belief that oneself is inherently flawed (Tracy & Robins, 2006).

Prevalence

As mentioned, guilt is a common human reaction. Everyone will likely experience at least mild guilt at some point in their life. It's when guilt morphs into shame that it becomes maladaptive. A national study of adults age 18 years and older found that the prevalence of maladaptive guilt was about 10% (Luck & Luck-Sikorski, 2021). In a separate study of children ages 9–10 years, the prevalence of maladaptive guilt was about 18% (Donohue et al., 2020). Guilt is often linked to depression (see Chapter Five). In one study, guilt was associated with depression almost 40% of the time (Luck & Luck-Sikorski, 2021).

Potential E-PFA Recommendations
(Think About Trying This)

What should Jasmine say to Andrew when they meet for lunch? What would you say if you were in Jasmine's position or a similar one? Listed below are the core aspects of our model.

1) Introduce yourself (if applicable), offer to help, set expectations, de-escalate (if needed).
2) Gather information. (*What happened? What hurts? How bad is it?*)
3) Clarify. (*What's the worst part of this?*)
4) Provide assistance. (*What do you need right now? How can I help?*)
   a. *Can Jasmine use problem-focused assistance?*
   b. *Can Jasmine use emotion-focused assistance?*
   c. *Can Jasmine use stress management?*
5) Make a plan. (*Next steps?*)

Introduce Yourself, Offer to Help, Set Expectations

- E–PFA begins with Jasmine "showing up," expressing a calm, nonconfrontational concern, and letting Andrew know she wants to help, not judge. And if she can't help, she will assist him in finding the help he needs. No introduction is necessary because they both know each other.

Gather Information

- Jasmine can encourage Andrew to talk about what he is experiencing. More specifically, she can ask him what the guilt feels like to him, how it's showing up in his life, and when it started. She can also ask how bad it's gotten, including whether it's interfering with work or outside activities. (*What happened? What hurts? How bad is it?*)

Clarify

- The goal of the clarification phase for Jasmine is to help her understand the nature of Andrew's feelings of guilt. A simple paraphrase — "Sounds like your son's graduation has triggered a wave of guilt and regret" — might be helpful.
- Jasmine can then seek greater specificity by asking, "As you think about this, Andrew, what's the worst part of it for you?"

Provide Assistance

- Jasmine can ask Andrew what he needs in that moment, or simply ask how she can help. But perhaps more directive assistance would be more effective. Remembering that E-PFA is not individualized psychotherapy, Jasmine can use a simplified checklist approach that applies to virtually all guilt reactions, regardless of their origin. The determination of responsibility or culpability typically falls into three categories: no true responsibility, partial responsibility, and complete responsibility. These are reviewed below.

Problem-Focused

- First, Jasmine should determine culpability. She can ask Andrew if he is truly responsible for the perceived neglect of his family. In this case it seems that he is, especially in light of the affair that contributed to his divorce. Sometimes, however, we accept responsibility because we want to believe we can control all the adversities in our lives, or because it's what we or others expect. If Andrew were not truly responsible, Jasmine could gently point that out; in other words, she could raise reasonable doubt. For example, if other factors contributed to the divorce, she could respectfully mention them. But she should avoid arguing or rushing to make excuses for Andrew.
- In Andrew's case, taking responsibility clearly seems warranted. But in a different situation, Jasmine could ask if Andrew believes he is 100% responsible. Nothing happens in a vacuum. Mistakes and wrongdoings are often the result of interacting factors.

Emotion-Focused

- If Jasmine determines that the guilt is warranted and Andrew is fully or mostly culpable, she might encourage him to "own it." Perhaps apologies are in order. For example, Jasmie could encourage Andrew to have conversations with his ex-wife and children about what he can do to improve things within the family, with the understanding that he can never erase what's occurred.
- Reminding Andrew of the words of acclaimed writer, poet, and civil rights activist Maya Angelou may help him manage his guilt, regret, and shame: "If I had known better, I would have done better." Tomorrow is a new day. It's the first day of the rest of your life. Do better!

Stress Management–Focused

- To help Andrew cope with the distress and guilt he's experiencing, Jasmine could ask how he has managed sadness and stress in the past, and what might help him cope better now. (*What has worked in the past to manage stress?*)

Make a Plan

- Jasmine can help Andrew make a plan to support his family, if possible, while also emphasizing the importance of forgiving himself. Encouraging Andrew to pursue individual or even family counseling might be an appropriate next step. (*Next steps?*)
- Jasmine might also help Andrew develop a stress management or resilience plan to navigate this period, including offering to follow up to get him started, while still encouraging professional support.

E-PFA Dialogue (It Might Sound Like This)

ANDREW (ARRIVING AT THE DESIGNATED LUNCH SPOT CLOSE TO FIFTEEN MINUTES LATE): I'm sorry for being late, Jasmine. I had trouble wrapping up an international call. Again, my apologies. Thank you so much for your willingness to meet with me.

JASMINE: I'll do all I can to help, Andrew. And if I'm not the best person to assist you, I'll certainly try to find you the help you need.

ANDREW: That sounds good. I appreciate you reaching out to me. Also, it's not lost on me that I want to talk with you about feeling guilty . . . and here I am feeling guilty about showing up late to meet with you. Again, my apologies.

JASMINE: It happens in our business—an occupational hazard, I guess. So, what's going on with you? You seemed distressed yesterday and mentioned several reasons about why you were feeling guilty.

ANDREW: My son's high school graduation is tonight. I really am so proud of all he's accomplished. But instead of being filled with great memories and feeling happy, it's completely dawned on me how much guilt and regret I have for messing up so much over the past 18 years — focusing too much on my professional life, the affair, neglecting my wife and kids.

JASMINE: When did these feelings of guilt and regret start?

ANDREW: It seems like they started, and then came crashing down, last week, after my ex-wife, Carla, called me. She said she felt the need to remind me that our son's graduation was coming up. She was concerned I might have forgotten, had a dinner meeting I couldn't miss, or even an overseas business trip scheduled.

JASMINE: How did you interpret her call?

ANDREW: I know what you might be thinking, and even though what Carla said to me might sound confrontational, I didn't think she was trying to be. She genuinely seemed to want to make sure I knew, probably because I've missed so many birthdays, soccer games, swim meets, plays, holidays, you name it. I think she just wanted to give me the chance to make it to this one. I truly appreciate that she called. But after I hung up the phone, I felt so incredibly sorry that she thought she had to remind me. And then the guilt took over, and I felt awful.

JASMINE: Let me ask, what does the guilt feel like to you?

ANDREW: Like I'm suffocating. I keep thinking about how much I've disappointed the people in my life that clearly should have meant the most to me.

JASMINE: How bad is it? Is it interfering with your work or outside activities?

ANDREW: By the end of last week, I started canceling meetings—and I never cancel meetings. I was so preoccupied with these thoughts and feelings, I knew I couldn't be at my best. I even stopped going to the exercise class I've been doing for the past two years when I'm home. These feelings have also been keeping me up at night when I'm trying to sleep.

JASMINE: I'm sorry you're experiencing this, Andrew. It sounds like your son's graduation has triggered a wave of guilt and regret.

ANDREW: Whew, you can say that again!

JASMINE: As you're thinking about this, what's the worst part?

ANDREW: Hmm . . . the feelings that I have are bad, that's for sure. But I think the worst part is that I can't take any of it back or do it over again. For all the so-called success I supposedly have, I feel like a total failure. Carla was absolutely justified in asking for a divorce. I own this. I was traveling constantly and totally ignored my family.

JASMINE: Those times we traveled together to meetings in Europe, I clearly remember you telling me how Carla and your two sons were doing. You always made it a point to bring something back for each of them from every trip. That doesn't sound like total neglect to me.

ANDREW: Okay, maybe not total neglect. But enough for Carla to rightfully ask for a divorce. And, of course, the affair!

JASMINE: Were there other factors that could have been involved? Now, I'm in no way trying to discount what you're saying. I'm just asking if there could have been some other, additional reasons for the divorce.

ANDREW: I appreciate you slowing me down and encouraging me to take a step back. But no, this is on me!

JASMINE: So maybe the best thing I can encourage you to do is to own your part in it—to own your stuff!

ANDREW (NODS THOUGHTFULLY AND REFLECTS FOR A FEW SECONDS): What should I do then?

JASMINE: Perhaps apologies are in order. It's never too late to try and make things better. Maybe you can talk with Carla and then have a conversation with your sons about what you can do moving forward to be a better father, while understanding that you can never erase what happened?

ANDREW: You're probably right.

JASMINE: Let me ask, Andrew, what have you done in the past to help yourself cope with feelings of sadness and stress? And any thoughts of what you can do now?

ANDREW: Well, I typically exercise, which I can start doing tomorrow. Also, I haven't found time to do so recently, but reading for pleasure brings me a lot of relief.

JASMINE: That sounds like a good plan. And speaking of plans, let's talk about how you can arrange times to have a conversation with Carla and visit the boys. Just as important, though, is working on forgiving yourself.

ANDREW: I appreciate all this, Jasmine. You're a good friend and colleague. I just hope it helps.

JASMINE: So, exercising and having conversations with Carla and the boys—sounds like a pretty good plan to help you through this. And just know I'm always available to talk more. Something else to consider, Andrew, is seeking some professional support. What you're describing seems like something that's been building for a while, and having someone to help you work through it could really make a difference.

ANDREW: I was thinking of this, Jasmine, and I'm glad you brought it up. It means a lot—feels validating.

JASMINE: If you feel comfortable, please let me know in the next couple of days how things go?

ANDREW: Will do. Now let's order. I want to get back to the office and finish up some things before the ceremony tonight. I 100% guarantee that I'll be there on time.

References

Cyberbullying Research Center. (2024). *2023 cyberbullying data.* https://cyberbullying.org/2023-cyberbullying-data

Donohue, M. R., Tillman, R., Perino, M. T., Whalen, D. J., Luby, J., & Barch, D. M. (2020). Prevalence and correlates of maladaptive guilt in middle childhood. *Journal of Affective Disorders, 263,* 64–71. https://doi.org/10.1016/j.jad.2019.11.075

Luck, T., & Luck-Sikorski, C. (2021). Feelings of guilt in the general adult population: Prevalence, intensity and association with depression. *Psychology, Health and Medicine, 26*(9), 1143–1153. https://doi.org/10.1080/13548506.2020.1859558

Luck, T., & Luck-Sikorski, C. (2022). The wide variety of reasons for feeling guilty in adults: Findings from a large cross-sectional web-based survey. *BMC Psychology, 10*(1), 198. https://doi.org/10.1186/s40359-022-00908-3

Tracy, J. L., & Robins, R. W. (2006). Appraisal antecedents of shame and guilt: Support for a theoretical model. *Personality and Social Psychology Bulletin, 32*(10), 1339–1351. https://doi.org/10.1177/0146167206290212

FIFTEEN | Grief

LUIS IS ATTENDING THE FUNERAL of the daughter of one of his closest friends, Miguel. Callista was only 18 years old when she died from a rare but aggressive form of cancer. After the funeral, Luis and about 30 other people go to Miguel's home. Luis sees his friend alone, crying in an adjacent room. He approaches Miguel to ask if there is anything he can do. Miguel thanks him for being there but replies no.

A week later, Luis decides to check in. He calls Miguel and asks if he can come over; Miguel agrees. Luis pulls up to the house and knocks on the door. Miguel, looking despondent and tired, answers with a quick, forced smile, and in a quiet voice invites Luis inside. What should Luis do?

What Is Grief?

Grief is the cognitive, emotional, and behavioral response to loss. Related terms include "bereavement," which refers to the objective fact of the loss, and "mourning," which refers to the public or social expression of grief (Stroebe et al., 2008). Mourning and grief strongly influence each other and are both strongly influenced by religious and cultural beliefs, particularly those related to death.

While most people associate grief with the loss of a loved one, including pets, through death, it can also result from other types of loss. For example, grief can be associated with more tangible losses, such as loss of a home, job, marriage, or physical ability due to injury or illness. It can arise from symbolic or abstract losses, such as the loss of faith, trust, hopes and dreams, self-esteem or honor, or a sense of control. Grief can even occur in an anticipation of a loss.

Several notable theories explore the process of grief. Erich Lindemann (1944), a prominent psychiatrist, studied grief in the aftermath of a nightclub fire in Boston on November 28, 1942, that resulted in the deaths of 492 people. He proposed that the tasks of grief and recovery entail:

- removal of a strong connection to the deceased;
- readjustment to the environment without the deceased;
- forming new relationships.

Most famously, Elisabeth Kübler-Ross (1969), a Swiss psychiatrist, described five stages of grief:

1) Denial and isolation
2) Anger
3) Bargaining
4) Depression
5) Acceptance

It is important to note that this model was not intended to represent a uniform, step-by-step progression through bereavement. In fact, there is minimal evidence that individuals pass through these stages in order.

In 1980, psychiatrist John Bowlby outlined four stages of grief:

1) Numbness (shock and intense distress)
2) Yearning and searching (lasting from months to years)
3) Disorganization and despair (as the loss becomes more "real," there is less yearning and more attempts to restructure)
4) Reorganization (accepting a new "normal")

More recently, William Worden (2018), a psychologist who has studied life-threatening illness and behavior for more than 45 years, developed a task-based theory of mourning, contrasting with previous "stage" theories of grief. His four tasks of mourning are:

1) Accepting the reality of the loss
2) Working through the physical and emotional pain
3) Adjusting to the new environment that no longer includes the deceased
4) Emotionally relocating, but not forgetting, the deceased and moving on

Again, these theories, along with their accompanying stages and tasks, are not intended to be prescriptive or diagnostic. Instead, for those providing PFA, they offer an overview of relevant concepts that one might encounter.

Key Features: Signs and Symptoms

The early stages of grief, referred to as acute grief, can be intensely painful and evoke behaviors and emotions that are atypical in everyday functioning, such as:

- Uncontrollable crying
- Avoidance

- Preoccupation with the deceased
- Shock
- Sadness
- Anger (see Chapter Nine)
- Pain
- Guilt (see Chapter Fourteen)
- Fear (see Chapter Seven)
- Hostility
- Irritability
- Yearning
- Intrusive images (see Chapter Eleven)
- Depersonalization (an out-of-body experience) (see Chapters Eleven and Seventeen)
- Being overwhelmed

In a description of the first year of the bereavement process, Bonanno and Kaltman (2001) suggest that most individuals will experience four types of grief symptoms:

1) *Cognitive disorganization*—difficulty comprehending or accepting the loss, which might include preoccupation, challenges with decision-making, making mistakes, or believing something is wrong with them. It also includes a sense that a part of them is missing, uncertainty about the future, and a search for meaning.

2) *Dysphoria*—a general sense of feeling uneasy, unhappy, despondent, "down in the dumps," and distressed. Other features include some of the symptoms noted above, such as pining or yearning and loneliness, which can be differentiated into social loneliness (not engaging in social activities) and emotional loneliness (a deeper sense of inner aloneness).

3) *Health deficits*—increased somatic problems (e.g., heart palpations, shortness of breath, loss of appetite, insomnia, compromised immune functioning). In a study conducted more than

60 years ago, Parkes (1964) reported that doctor visits in the first six months after the death of a spouse increased by 60%. Conversely, Prigerson and others (2001) found that women who had been bereaved for about four months and reported high levels of grief were less likely to seek health services, despite experiencing significant health issues, such as functional impairment or high blood pressure. There have also been long-standing associations between the death of a loved one and increased mortality of the bereaved person. In fact, King and colleagues (2017) reported that this risk was greatest during the first three months after the loss. Another study has shown that those experiencing bereavement due to a loved one's death by suicide have rates of suicidal ideation (see Chapter Sixteen) ranging from 14.1% to 49% (Molina et al., 2019).

4) *Disrupted social and occupational functioning* — often seen as social withdrawal and isolation, as well difficulty keeping up with occupational and social tasks. This may manifest in challenges managing work demands and spare time, as well as difficulties cultivating new relationships.

The Course of Grief

Despite what many people believe, there is no specific time frame or typical course for grief. One's experience of grief is shaped by the event, the individual characteristics of the bereaved person, and the assistance they receive. As Shakespeare aptly wrote, "Everyone can master grief, but he who has it." Everyone grieves differently, and there is no right or wrong way to grieve. As mentioned earlier, grief does not follow a linear progression and it is not a fixed state; rather, it's a process that starts, stops, comes, and goes.

Despite the individual nature of grief, it is generally accepted that most bereaved individuals are resilient. Although they may experience initial distress symptoms, they tend to improve after about six months. Most can attain a sense of acceptance, maintain productivity at work, and even find meaning in the loss (Bonnano, 2004). Many researchers believe that most symptoms of grief fully resolve in one to two years. In fact, a recent study assessing the trajectory of grief found that within about two years:

- 66.4% of the sample exhibited resilience,
- 25.1% exhibited chronic elevated grief, and
- 8.4% showed significant reductions or recovery in grief symptoms.

The last group was similar to the chronic group through 6 months postbereavement, but by 12–15 months, they resembled the resilient group (Djelantik et al., 2022).

It is important to understand that even though most people appear to recover in 12–24 months, and professional assistance can usually support that process, acute distress or a crisis can arise at any point, regardless of the time since the actual loss, and may still benefit from E-PFA.

Complicated/Prolonged Grief

Notwithstanding the evidence that most people are resilient after a serious loss, data suggest that some individuals may experience more intense grief reactions that last longer than expected. Those experiencing a combination of intensity and duration (lasting well beyond six months), with symptoms, such as intense yearning, that become the focus of their lives and impair daily functioning, are considered to have prolonged or complicated grief (Shear, 2015). While prolonged and intense grief reactions can occur following the loss of any close, meaningful relationship, they seem particularly pronounced for parents following the death of their child, or in cases where the death is sudden or violent (Lobb, 2010).

Posttraumatic Growth

Despite the primary focus on the negative symptoms associated with grieving, there appear to be positive aspects for many of those who experience a serious loss or life crisis. This view is based on the premise that adversity can unintentionally produce constructive changes in how one views themselves, others, and the world in general. The transformation is referred to as posttraumatic growth (Tedeschi & Calhoun, 1995). For example, as early as two months after a loss, a study showed that 42% of the bereaved respondents said they were better people for having experienced the loss (Shuchter & Zisook, 1993). Tedeschi and Calhoun (1996) developed the Post-Traumatic Growth Inventory, a measure that assesses positive responses in the following areas:

- New possibilities
- Relating to others
- Personal strength
- Spirituality change
- Appreciation of life

Potential E-PFA Recommendations
(Think About Trying This)

What should Luis say to Miguel? What would you say if you were in Luis's position or one similar?

The general E-PFA intervention remains fundamentally the same as we have seen in other chapters.

1) Introduce yourself (if applicable), offer to help, set expectations, de-escalate (if needed).
2) Gather information. (*What happened? What hurts? How bad is it?*)
3) Clarify. (*What's the worst part?*)
4) Provide assistance. (*What do you need right now? How can I help?*)
   a. *Can Luis use problem-focused assistance?*
   b. *Can Luis use emotion-focused assistance?*
   c. *Can Luis use stress management?*
5) Make a plan. (*Next steps?*)

Introduce Yourself, Offer to Help, Set Expectations, De-escalate

- In instances of grief, E-PFA begins with "showing up" while emitting a calm, supportive presence.

Gather Information

- Luis can ask Miguel to talk about what he is experiencing. (*What hurts?*) There is no need to review the details of his daughter's death, unless Miguel wants to discuss them. (*What happened?*)
- Luis must take care not to probe too deeply in this circumstance.
- Luis can ask Miguel if he is able to accomplish the things he needs to do on a daily basis, but it's important to adjust expectations in terms how much time has passed since the funeral. (*How bad is it?*)

Clarify

- Minimal paraphrasing may be useful, but in some instances none is necessary.
- Sometimes asking what the "worst part" of what Miguel is going through can be useful, as it would give Luis direction on how he might better assist his friend.

Provide Assistance

- Luis can consider asking open-ended questions, such as, "What do you need most right now?" and "How can I help?" Sometimes these questions are all that is needed. If necessary, and as appropriate, Luis can be more directive in his questioning, using examples from one or more of the approaches suggested below. That said, a general caution must be made against doing too much when attempting to assist someone in grief.

Problem-Focused

- Luis should be very careful not to try to "solve" the problem. As hard as it may be to believe, we've heard comments like, "You can still have more children," or, in the case of losing a spouse, "You can always remarry." Needless to say, such comments, while well-intended, can come across as dismissive and hurtful. There is no way to solve the loss of a loved one. Other types of losses, however, may have resolutions.
- While Luis cannot solve the problem, he can help mitigate Miguel's loss. One of the most effective ways to do this is by finding ways to honor the person or thing that has been lost. Many worthwhile initiatives (e.g., cancer screening, drunk driving prevention programs) and even nonprofit foundations have been created in the wake of loss.
- One of the most effective ways to assist with grief, and something Luis might consider, is helping people channel the energy consumed by grief into something productive, whatever that may be.

Emotion-Focused

- In some instances, comments may be made that do not attempt to solve or mitigate the problem itself, but rather to lessen the acute suffering. Luis should avoid comments that begin with the phrase "At least" because they are usually intended to shift the focus to what the bereaved person still has rather than what they have lost. While these comments come from a sincere desire to help, they can be remarkably insensitive. Gratitude can help reduce acute distress, but timing is critical. In Miguel's case, such an approach might be premature.

Stress Management–Focused

- To help Miguel cope with the stress of loss and grief, Luis can ask him how he has handled sadness and stress in the past, and what might help him now. It is important for Luis to recognize that the anguish of grief is unique. The intensity of the emptiness or void Miguel feels will probably be unparalleled for him, but basic stress management and wellness practices can still be effective in easing the pain.

Make a Plan

- Luis can help Miguel make a plan to move forward, especially if Miguel is open to ideas for self-care.
- He might suggest that Miguel join a support group or pursue counseling. But again, timing is essential. That which is rejected today may be an effective intervention tomorrow.

E-PFA Dialogue (It Might Sound Like This)

MIGUEL: Thank you for coming over. Do you want something to drink?

LUIS: No, thank you. I'm simply here for you.

MIGUEL: That means a lot.

LUIS: I will do whatever you need, Miguel. I'll just sit here if you'd like.

MIGUEL: I've been doing a lot of sitting, thinking, and talking to myself this past week. Having you here now is probably good for me.

LUIS: I'm following your lead. But let me ask, are you okay to talk about what happened?

MIGUEL (PAUSING): It's been really rough, but yeah. I'm good talking with you.

LUIS: What, if anything, would you like to share with me about what you're experiencing?

MIGUEL (AFTER 30 SECONDS OF SILENCE): Why? . . . Why, Luis? Why? It's not fair! She had her whole life in front of her. She was a perfect child, an angel! Why her? Why not me? I've lived long enough. And to watch how she suffered at the end—no parent should have to witness that.

LUIS: I am so sorry, Miguel.

MIGUEL (AFTER MORE SILENCE): But I was there for her. My wife, Sarah, and I . . . we were there for her, through all of it.

LUIS: It must have been so unbelievably challenging for you and Sarah. Again, I am so sorry, Miguel. I'm here to listen. You can discuss as many or as few of the details as you'd like.

MIGUEL: It was how the cancer took her. It was awful . . . just awful. I don't want to say any more about it now.

LUIS: I understand. It sounds just horrible. I appreciate you sharing as much as you're comfortable with, Miguel. It seems like there were a lot of really bad parts.

MIGUEL: You know, one of the worst parts, and I was thinking of this earlier today, is not being able to walk her down the aisle on her wedding day. Luis, how am I ever going to be able to get over this? I'm a problem-solver. How do I solve this?

LUIS: I'm sorry, Miguel. I genuinely wish there was some type of formula to help fix this. But there's no such thing as solving the loss of a loved one. It's so unfair.

MIGUEL: I get that, I really do. But then, what are some options? How can I make any sense out of this terrible situation?

LUIS: I was thinking of this on my way over. Sometimes, finding a way to honor the memory of someone you've lost can help ease the pain a little.

MIGUEL: Like what?

LUIS: Well, I'm thinking of organizations like Mothers Against Drunk Driving or the Amy Winehouse Foundation. They both work to make a positive difference, like preventing substance abuse. And they also honor the memory of someone who died.

MIGUEL (AFTER SEVERAL SECONDS OF SILENCE): Okay . . . I see. I remember how much Callista used to love volunteering at clothes drives to help kids in need. She used to light up when she was able to deliver the most boxes. Maybe we could start something like that in her name?

LUIS: Hmm . . . Clothes from Callista. Why not?

MIGUEL: Something to think about. But it won't take the pain away, and it won't bring her back.

LUIS: You're absolutely right, Miguel. It won't. But maybe in time it might be something that brings you solace and a way to remember her.

MIGUEL: I'm just trying to get through each day, sometime each hour, or even just each minute.

LUIS: I know there's probably no pain that comes close to what you're going through now. And there probably never will be.

Grief is unique. The emptiness, the void—it's overwhelming. But you've gotten through tough times before. What's helped you cope then?

MIGUEL: Support . . . and family. As you know, I'm an outgoing person. My sleep is off, and I'm not eating regularly. I've been having headaches, which could be from a lot of things. I know I'm not drinking enough water.

LUIS: Sounds like some basis stress management techniques can help. Making sure you eat regularly and stay hydrated can take a slight edge off your physical discomfort. Taking a walk, getting outside every day can be beneficial too.

MIGUEL: All things I should be doing. I'll need to keep reminding myself, but it's so hard to go through this.

LUIS: I can only imagine, Miguel. But you won't be going through this alone. I'm a five-minute drive away and can be here as much or as little as you like.

MIGUEL: I know you will, and I know that you'll do your best to try and understand. That's what makes you such a good friend.

LUIS: While I might not be able to fully understand, there are those out there who do.

MIGUEL: What do you mean?

LUIS: Something to consider, if and when you're ready, is a support group for people who have experienced a loss like yours. It might not feel right today or tomorrow or anytime relatively soon, but it might be helpful in the future.

MIGUEL: I'll talk it over with Sarah. This has been without a doubt the most awful experience of my life, but I am grateful for you, Luis.

References

Bonanno, G. A. (2004). Loss, trauma, and human resilience: Have we underestimated the human capacity to thrive after extremely aversive events? *American Psychologist, 59*(1), 20–28. https://doi.org/10.1037/0003-066X.59.1.20

Bonanno, G. A., & Kaltman, S. (2001). The varieties of grief experience. *Clinical Psychology Review, 21*(5), 705–734. https://doi.org/10.1016/S0272-7358(00)00062-3

Bowlby, J. (1980). *Loss: Sadness and depression. Attachment and loss* (Vol. 3). Basic Books.

Djelantik, A. A. A. M., Robinaugh, D. J., & Boelen, P. A. (2022). The course of symptoms in the first 27 months following bereavement: A latent trajectory analysis of prolonged grief, posttraumatic stress, and depression. *Psychiatry Research, 311*, 114472. https://doi.org/10.1016/j.psychres.2022.114472

King, M., Lodwick, R., Jones, R., Whitaker, H., & Petersen, I. (2017). Death following partner bereavement: A self-controlled case series analysis. *PLOS One*. https://doi.org/10.1371/journal.prone.0173870

Kübler-Ross, E. (1969). *On death and dying: What the dying have to teach doctors, nurses, clergy and their own families.* Macmillan Publishing.

Lindemann, E. (1944). Symptomatology and management of acute grief. *American Journal of Psychiatry, 101*(2), 141–148. https://doi.org/10.1176/ajp.101.2.141

Lobb, E. A., Kristjanson, L. J., Aoun, S. M., Monterosso, L., Halkett, G. K. B., & Davies, A. (2010). Predictors of complicated grief: A systematic review of empirical studies. *Death Studies, 34*(8), 673–698. https://doi.org/10.1080/07481187.2010.496686

Molina, N., Viola, M., Rogers, M., Ouyang, D., Gang, J., Derry, H., & Prigerson, H. G. (2019). Suicidal ideation in bereavement: A systematic review. *Behavioral Sciences, 9*, 53. https://doi.org/10.3390/bs9050053

Parkes, C. M. (1964). Effects of bereavement on physical and mental health: A study of the medical records of widows. *British Medical Journal, 2*(5404), 274–279. https://doi.org/10.1136/bmj.2.5404.274

Prigerson, H., Silverman, G. K., Jacobs, S., Maciejewski, P., Kasl, S. V., & Rosenheck, R. (2001). Traumatic grief, disability and the underutilization of health services: A preliminary look. *Primary Psychiatry, 8*, 61–69.

Shear, M. K. (2015). Complicated grief. *New England Journal of Medicine,* 372(2), 153–160. https://doi.org/10.1056/NEJMcp1315618

Shuchter, S., & Zisook, S. (1993). The course of normal grief. In M. S. Stroebe, W. Stroebe, & R. O. Hansson (Eds.), *Handbook of bereavement: Theory, research and intervention* (pp. 23–43). Cambridge University Press.

Stroebe, M. S., Hansson, R. O., Schut, H., & Stoebe, W. (2008). Bereavement research: Contemporary perspectives. In M. S. Stroebe, H. Hansson, W. Schut, & W. Stroebe (Eds.), *Handbook of bereavement research and practice: 21st century perspectives* (pp. 3–25). American Psychological Association Press. https://doi.org/10.1037/14498001

Tedeschi, R. G., & Calhoun, L. G. (1995). *Trauma and transformation: Growing in the aftermath of suffering.* Sage.

Tedeschi, R. G., & Calhoun, L. G. (1996). The Posttraumatic Growth Inventory: Measuring the positive legacy of trauma. *Journal of Traumatic Stress,* 9(3), 455–471. https://doi.org/10.1007/BF02103658

Worden, W. (2018). *Grief counseling and grief therapy: A handbook for the mental health practitioner* (5th ed.). Springer Nature.

SIXTEEN | Suicidal Thoughts

AIDEN IS A 19-YEAR-OLD COLLEGE STUDENT ap-
proaching the end of his first academic year at a university
located on a rural campus about 200 miles from his home. He
is currently a premed major and did well academically in
his first semester. Socially, however, he just doesn't seem to
fit in. Even Aiden would admit that he feels awkward in so-
cial settings. At the encouragement of his roommate, Marcus,
Aiden attended several social events on campus, but he left
early each time after attracting ridicule from other students.
That ridicule has spilled over onto social media, where it has
escalated into bullying.

Aiden's parents have encouraged him to "tough it out," but
he says he no longer has the energy to do so. His grades have
begun to suffer this spring semester. He recently confided in
Marcus that he has been feeling depressed and does not want
to leave his dorm room for fear of being bullied again.

Two days after that conversation, Aiden was bullied in
the dining hall and returned to his room without finishing
his meal. Marcus came back about 30 minutes later, unaware

of what had happened, and found Aiden sitting at the kitchen table, gazing at the wall. When Marcus asked what was going on, Aiden replied that it was the last day he would have to tolerate the bullying. Marcus encouraged him to ignore the bullies, but Aiden responded, "You don't understand. I can't take it anymore. I'm going to kill myself tonight."

What Are Suicidal Thoughts?

Suicidal thoughts and feelings, referred to as suicidal ideation, entail imagining, thinking about, planning, or even mentally rehearsing the act of suicide. The feelings associated with these thoughts often include hopelessness, despair, being a burden, and psychological pain. While some people have passive suicidal ideation, where they think about death, not being around, or not wanting to wake up but have no intention to act on these thoughts, others might have active suicidal ideation, where they may create a plan and intend to take action to see it through. Suicide, then, is seeing it through or the intentional act of ending one's own life.

Key Features and Risk Factors

Suicidal thoughts and actions typically do not arise spontaneously, although the actions themselves can sometimes be impulsive. These thoughts and actions—including self-injurious actions without intention to die—arise from feelings of desperation, hopelessness, and helplessness. In rare cases, they may also be driven by a desire to exact revenge through self-harm or self-destruction.

The World Health Organization (WHO) (2024b) highlights the global link between suicide and mental health disorders, in particular alcohol use (see Chapter Thirteen) and depression (see Chapter Five). However, WHO also notes that many suicides can occur impulsively in reaction to stressors such as financial problems, relationship issues, chronic physical or emotional pain, and illness.

Evidence for the impulsive nature of suicide comes from a study of 82 suicide-attempt survivors, in which 48% reported that the time between their initial thought of suicide and the actual attempt was 10 minutes or less (Deisenhammer et al., 2009). Similarly, a study of 153 survivors of nearly lethal attempts between the ages of 13 and 34 years found that 24% spent less than 5 minutes between deciding to attempt suicide and the attempt itself, and 5% reported a gap of just about 1 second. In the same study, males were almost twice as likely as females to attempt suicide impulsively, with such attempts most commonly occurring between 7:01 p.m. and 6:59 a.m. (Simon et al., 2001).

The WHO (2024b) also notes that experiencing a disaster, violence, abuse, or loss is associated with increased risk of suicidal behavior. Worldwide, rates are particularly high among vulnerable populations such as refugees, indigenous people, prisoners, and lesbian, gay, bisexual, transgender, and intersex (LGBTI) persons. In the United States, non-Hispanic American Indian/Alaska Native individuals have the highest suicide risk, followed by non-Hispanic white people. According to the CDC (2023), other at-risk groups in the United States include military veterans, people living in rural areas, and those employed in high-risk occupations like mining and construction. Consistent with global data, young people in the United States who identify as LGBTI are also at increased of suicidal thoughts and behaviors, particularly if they are in an unsupportive environment.

Suicidal thoughts sometimes arise after the onset of a life-changing or terminal illness. They may also emerge after the development of a disability. But it's worth noting that physical factors are typically triggers—not essential causes—of suicidal thoughts.

Physiologically, suicidal thoughts have been associated with low levels of serotonin, elevated levels of adrenocorticotropic hormone, elevated cortisol, and neuroinflammatory processes. Decreased activity in the brain's prefrontal cortex has also been observed—an important finding, as this region of the brain is responsible for rational thought.

Prevalence

The prevalence of suicidal thoughts is difficult to accurately measure, but according to the CDC, in the United States, 13.6% of adults aged 18–25 years and 22% of high school students reported having serious thoughts of suicide in 2023 (CDC 2023).

Death by suicide remains a staggering global public health issue. According to the WHO (2023):

- More than 703,000 people die by suicide every year.
- Suicide is the fourth leading cause of death globally among 15- to 29-year-olds.
- Death by suicide accounts for 1.3% of all deaths worldwide.
- Ingestion of pesticides, mostly in rural agricultural areas in low and middle-income countries, is estimated to be the cause of death in 20% of global suicides.

In the United States, according to the CDC (2023):

- There were 49,449 deaths by suicide in 2022.
- This equates to one death every 11 minutes.
- Firearms were used in more than 50% of US suicides, followed by suffocation (26%) and then poisoning (12%), which includes overdosing on medication.

Worldwide, more than twice as many males die by suicide as females (WHO, 2021). In the United States, the disparity is even greater: Males make up 50% of the population but account for nearly 80% of suicide deaths (CDC, 2023).

As troubling as these numbers are, the WHO (2024a) estimates that, for every completed suicide, there are likely more than 20 attempts. A suicide attempt is defined as someone harming themselves with any intent to end their life. In the United States in 2022, more than 1.7 million adults attempted suicide (CDC, 2023).

Warning Signs for Suicide Attempts

In addition to these broad epidemiologic data on suicide, it is important to recognize behavioral warning signs — sometimes called lethality factors — that increase the risk of a completed suicide, such as:

- Previous suicide attempt(s)
- History of impulsive acts
- Making passive statements, such as talking about wishing they hadn't been born, or hoping to go to sleep and not wake up
- Discussing active wishes to harm themselves (which should be taken more seriously than the passive statements described above)
- Withdrawal from social contact
- Hopelessness, feeling like giving up
- Increased agitation or mood swings
- Increased use of alcohol or drugs
- Changes in routine (e.g., sleeping a lot more)
- Saying goodbye to people
- Acquiring the means for suicide (e.g., purchasing a gun or pills)
- Improvement of mood (possibly due to a sense of relief from having made the decision, including date, time, and means)
- Giving away belongings

Remember that about half of suicide attempts with a high risk of death may be impulsive!

Recognizing that someone may be considering suicide can be chilling. While some individuals might display one or more of the signs listed above or openly talk about their thoughts, others may conceal their suicidal ideations and keep their intentions to themselves. This makes it almost impossible to know exactly what someone is thinking or planning. But if you suspect someone is thinking of suicide, it is better to confront the issue — possibly facing their discomfort or anger if you're wrong — than to ignore it.

Protective Factors That Might Reduce the Risk of Suicide

While the focus on suicide often centers around identifying risk factors, some researchers have highlighted the following factors that may reduce its likelihood (Gask & Morriss, 2008; Joiner et al., 2007):

- Availability of social support (see account of Kevin Hines in Chapter One)
- Affirmation that a specific event will prevent suicide (e.g., getting a job before the end of the month; reconciliation with a partner)
- Focusing on the future and anticipating upcoming events, both short- and long-term
- Fearing death, physical disfigurement, or permanent cognitive or emotional damage, all of which may generate ambivalence about death
- Worrying that the suicide attempt will have little impact on others, including family and friends
- Concern about leaving children or loved ones without care, feeling a sense of duty to family

- Strong religious beliefs
- Lack of access to intended means of suicide

Potential E-PFA Recommendations
(Think About Trying This)

E-PFA interventions with someone contemplating self-injury or suicide are likely to be among the most challenging situations a person may face. The recommendations below are offered as guidelines to help mitigate acute distress and connect the person with additional, protective care. They are not meant to serve as a formal or prescriptive course in suicide intervention. Formal, recognized suicide intervention requires more advanced training. The purpose here is to provide introductory insights and suggestions for responding to this serious situation—one that is best treated as a medical emergency.

The goals of intervention from this perspective are fourfold:

1) Interrupt the train of suicidal thoughts.
2) Reduce acute distress, if possible.
3) Prolong life by delaying any suicidal actions.
4) Prolong life by accessing some form of immediate protective care.

With these conditions noted, what can Marcus do to support Aiden in this situation? What would you do if you found yourself in a situation similar to Marcus's? Let's look at the scenario through the five-phase E-PFA lens, with the above goals in mind.

The general E-PFA structure remains fundamentally the same but is far more targeted:

1) Introduce yourself (if applicable), offer to help, set expectations, de-escalate (if needed).

2) Gather information. (*What happened? What hurts? How bad is it?*)

3) Clarify suicidal ideation.

4) Provide assistance. It is essential to interrupt suicidal thoughts and prevent self-injurious action through delay or distraction.

5) Make a plan to access protective support, and implement the plan. Protective care is always the final step in this approach.

Introduce Yourself, Offer to Help, Set Expectations

- PFA begins with Marcus "showing up," expressing a calm, non-confrontational concern, and letting Aiden know he wants to help, if possible. And if he can't help, he will assist Aiden in finding the help he needs.

- In the case of suicidal thoughts, it's imperative for Marcus to focus on interrupting the suicidal thinking and doing everything he can to prevent Aiden from acting on those thoughts until additional protective assistance is available. To do this effectively, Marcus should avoid arguing or saying anything provocative. He should also steer clear of an attempt at "reverse psychology" — for example, statements like "Well, just go ahead and kill yourself!" are dangerous and unhelpful. At the same time, Marcus cannot be dismissive; comments like, "Oh, you would never kill yourself!" can invalidate Aiden's feelings and shut down meaningful communication.

- Here are some additional considerations about suicidal thinking that Marcus should keep in mind before beginning his E-PFA intervention:

  - Marcus should offer to meet Aiden's basic needs (e.g., food or water).

  - He should be aware of his own personal safety (avoid putting himself at risk of harm).

- As much as possible given the circumstance, Marcus should speak in a calm and reassuring tone.
- He should try to reduce environmental stressors (e.g., other people watching, noise, bright sunlight).
- He needs to take seriously what Aiden is saying or implying.
- He should not leave Aiden alone, unless Marcus believes his own safety is directly threatened.
- He should recognize that Aiden is most likely not thinking flexibly and might have limited problem-solving capacity at the moment.
- Marcus should understand Aiden doesn't just need reassurances. What Marcus *can* reassure Aiden of is that he will get him help.
- Marcus shouldn't promise to keep their conversation confidential.
- Marcus should be open and ask Aiden direct questions like "Are you thinking about suicide?" or "Are you thinking of killing yourself?" It is a potentially harmful misconception that asking about suicide encourages it. In fact, many people who are suicidal feel relieved to talk about it (Gask & Morriss, 2008).
- Marcus can try to determine if Aiden is under the influence of alcohol or drugs (see Chapter Thirteen).
- Marcus's primary goal is to help Aiden choose to stay alive and to prevent or at least delay self-injurious actions. The longer the delay, the less likely an attempt becomes—at least in the immediate term.
- Marcus can enhance Aiden's hope and confidence.
- Again, Marcus's goal is to ensure that Aiden gets to the next level of care. This might mean calling emergency services (9-1-1 in the United States) and waiting for help to arrive, contacting the Suicide and Crisis Lifeline (9-8-8 in the United States), or helping Aiden get to the hospital.

Gather Information

- Marcus should encourage Aiden to talk about what he is experiencing. Asking questions like "What's going on?" can open up the conversation. When Aiden reveals that he is contemplating suicide, Marcus should guide him to express the feelings underlying those thoughts. Is Aiden feeling angry, hopeless, frustrated, or even vengeful? For example, Marcus might say, "Bullying is terrible, but what are you saying to yourself?" Or, "How do you feel when you are bullied?"

Clarify

- The goal of the clarification phase is for Marcus to clearly understand the nature of Aiden's thoughts and true intentions. It is essential for Marcus to ask Aiden a direct question such as, "Aiden, are you thinking about hurting yourself or killing yourself?" Or, "Aiden, are you considering dying by suicide?"

- If Aiden says yes, he is considering suicide, Marcus can follow up by asking about his intention. He could ask, "Aiden you sound desperate, but do you really want to die, or do you want to live differently?" — for example, to have the bullying end. Remember that the motivation for suicide is typically not a desire for death itself, but rather a desire to escape something else (e.g., bullying, emotional pain, physical pain, hopelessness, despair, financial problems).

- If Aiden's intention to harm or kill himself is clearly established, Marcus should assess the lethality of the situation. He should ask Aiden if he has thought about how or when he plans to carry out the act — in other words, "Do you have a plan?" It is important for Marcus to then determine whether Aiden has access to the means of carrying out the plan (e.g., a weapon, pills). Marcus should also ask Aiden if this is his *only* plan. Sometimes individuals who are suicidal may not disclose a well-thought-out plan unless asked directly, especially if they believe that the person with them genuinely cares and is interested in helping. Marcus should be cautious if Aiden mentions plans that involve avoiding detection (e.g., waiting for others to not be at home), because they might indicate a more serious intent.

Provide Assistance

- By being present and engaging in a supportive conversation, Marcus likely achieved his first goal of interrupting Aiden's obsessive suicidal thoughts. In many cases, people contemplating suicide do so because they feel out of control and see no other options, but they do not really want to die. The next step for Marcus is to help Aiden explore alternatives to suicide. This can be seen as a form of psychological or emotional pain management.
- Without arguing, Marcus can try to persuade Aiden that suicide is not the only solution, nor the best one, and that seeking help from others can be a more effective solution. It may be useful for Marcus to point out the potential unintended consequences of suicide that Aiden might not have considered. For example (Heard et al., 2022):
  - Suicide can create more problems than it solves.
  - Suicide is a permanent solution to what is usually a temporary problem.
  - Suicide does not always achieve the intended outcome.
  - Suicide creates the ripple effects of grief, guilt, and shame for friends and family.
  - Suicide can serve as a model for others to follow, potentially leading them to consider similar actions.
  - Suicide will often be how the person is remembered.

In the final analysis, Marcus's goal in using E-PFA is not to "cure" Aiden of his suicidal thoughts but to prolong Aiden's life. His focus should be on interrupting Aiden's action-oriented, obsessive suicidal thoughts, preventing or delaying self-injurious actions, and encouraging Aiden to accept protective support. Thus, "delaying" suicidal action, rather than eliminating suicidal thoughts altogether, becomes an acceptable outcome. Research shows that most people have second thoughts about suicide 24 to 48 hours after their first expression of intent (Cask & Morriss, 2008), so by delaying Aiden's actions, Marcus may have a lasting positive impact. In essence, Marcus is aiming to prevent Aiden from making a long-term decision to solve what is often a short-term problem.

Make a Plan

1) Exactly how Marcus enlists the aid of higher-level supportive and protective care will depend on how the situation evolves. Calling 9-1-1 or 9-8-8 to access emergency medical support is often the safest and most prudent default plan.

2) Marcus might also consider calling the dorm resident assistant and campus security for immediate assistance.

3) Gaining Aiden's active participation can be useful. For example, Marcus might say, "Aiden, I'm so sorry that things have reached this level. But don't let people who don't truly know or understand you control your happiness or your life. You need additional supportive care. Who should we call—the student resident coordinator, the campus hotline, or should I call 9-1-1 or 9-8-8?"

4) Once Aiden has conveyed to Marcus that he has seriously considered suicide, it's important that Aiden not be allowed to "take it back." Marcus must stay with Aiden and not leave until some form of protective care is in place.

E-PFA Dialogue (It Might Sound Like This)

MARCUS: I'm so sorry that things have gotten so bad for you, Aiden. I'm here to listen and to help you anyway I can. And if I can't help you, I promise I'll assist you in getting the help you need.

AIDEN: It's too late . . . I can't take this anymore.

MARCUS (AS CALMLY AS POSSIBLE): I want you to know that I hear exactly what you're saying. And I'm not going anywhere. *(Backing up a few feet to the refrigerator.)* I'm just going to get a bottle of water. Want one?

AIDEN: Huh?

MARCUS: A bottle of water?

AIDEN: Yeah, okay.

MARCUS (MAINTAINING VISUAL CONTACT WITH AIDEN, HANDS A BOTTLE TO HIM): What's going on?

AIDEN: The bullying happened again! I just wanted to eat dinner and be left alone. I left the dining hall, came back here, and have been staring at the wall thinking of ways to end it.

MARCUS: When you say "end it," Aiden, are you talking about ending your feelings related to the bullying?

AIDEN (PAUSING): . . . I guess I am.

MARCUS: Bullying is terrible—period. But what are you saying to yourself? How do you feel when you're bullied?

AIDEN: I feel weak, embarrassed, and inconsequential. I don't mean a thing to them . . . or probably anyone. While sitting here, I got frustrated and then so angry, partly at myself for believing I have no other choice but to take the bullying, but then I got pissed at them for being so callous and cruel. I wish

I had the strength to physically hurt them. Instead, I'm going to end this by hurting myself.

MARCUS: Aiden, you said this earlier, and just alluded to it again, but I want to make sure I'm clear on what your thoughts and intentions are. Are you thinking about killing yourself?

AIDEN (SILENT FOR 20 SECONDS): Yes.

MARCUS: I hear what you're saying, and I appreciate your honesty. I imagine that it can't be easy to tell me that. But, Aiden, do you really want to die, or is it that you want the bullying to end?

AIDEN: I want the despair and emotional pain to end. And I was thinking of how to do it before you came in.

MARCUS: Thinking of how to do it? Does this mean that you have a plan?

AIDEN: I don't have a weapon, so I was thinking of waiting for you to go to sleep, then I'd take the 20 or so acetaminophen capsules that I have in my room, drink the bottle of whiskey I got last week, and then, if I'm able, walk into traffic.

MARCUS: Whew! I'm not gonna lie. That's tough for me to hear, but again, I respect your honesty—and I'm glad you're talking to me. Let me ask . . . is this the only plan you have?

AIDEN (PAUSING): I haven't completely thought it through since I just realized I should do this . . . so, yeah, this is the only plan I have.

MARCUS (ATTEMPTING TO INTERRUPT AIDEN'S SUICIDAL THOUGHTS): Do you really want to die? Or, like I asked, do you want to live differently?

AIDEN: Live differently? I'm not sure I'm thinking too clearly. What do you mean?

MARCUS: The pain you're feeling from the bullying is real. Let's talk about other ways it can be handled without hurting yourself. Suicide is not the only option, and definitely not the best one. It would have a huge impact on your family and real friends, including me. And honestly, it's a permanent solution to an emotional problem that is short term. We can come up with other ways to help you feel more in control and get you through this. You don't have to go through it alone.

AIDEN: Are you trying to talk me out of it?

MARCUS: I'm listening to what you're saying, and I hear how serious this is for you. But you just said you weren't thinking too clearly. I know that dying by suicide is not how you want to be remembered, Aiden. And I'm even more certain that you should delay making any type of life-altering decision, especially this one, when you're not thinking clearly.

AIDEN: I'm feeling too vulnerable right now, Marcus. I can't make any promises. If you hadn't come in when you did, I might have already started the process.

MARCUS: Well, for whatever reason—and it might have been for us to have this conversation—I came back when I did. And I'm really glad I did. Aiden, I'm so sorry that things have reached this level. But don't give your happiness and control of your life to people who clearly don't know you and for some reason don't appreciate or understand you. I will stay with you, Aiden, but you need additional support. Think of it as psychological pain management. So, should we call the student resident coordinator, the campus hotline, or should I call 9-1-1 or 9-8-8?

AIDEN: You're not going to let this go, are you? You're going to make me do something.

MARCUS: Aiden, hurting yourself or ending your life would be the biggest decision you'd ever make. We both know people make bad decisions when they're under stress. This is a tough time for you. And I care too much, Aiden. You're worth it.

AIDEN (AFTER A PAUSE): Call the resident coordinator first.

MARCUS (DIALING HIS PHONE): I'm calling him now. And I'm not going anywhere until he arrives.

AIDEN: I hear ya.

References

Centers for Disease Control and Prevention. (2023). *Suicide data and statistics.* https://www.cdc.gov/suicide/suicide-data-statistics.html

Deisenhammer, E. A., Ing, C.-M., Strauss, R., Kemmler, G., Hinterhuber, H., & Weiss, E. M. (2009). The duration of the suicidal process: How much time is left for intervention between consideration and accomplishment of a suicide attempt? *Journal of Clinical Psychiatry, 70*(1), 19–24. https://doi.org/10.4088/JCP.07m03904

Gask, L., & Morriss, R. (2008). Assessment and immediate management of people at risk of harming themselves. *The Foundation Years, 4*(2), 64–68. https://doi.org/10.1016/j.mpfou.2008.02.007

Heard, T. R., McGill, K., Skehan, J., & Rose, B. (2022). The ripple effect, silence and powerlessness: Hidden barriers to discussing suicide in Australian aboriginal communities. *BMC Psychology, 10,* 23. https://doi.org/10.1186/s40359-022-00724-9

Joiner, T., Kalafat, J., Draper, J., Stokes, H., Knudson, M., Berman, A. L., & McKeon, R. (2007). Establishing standards for the assessment of suicide risk among callers to the National Suicide Prevention Lifeline. *Suicide and Life-Threatening Behavior, 37*(3), 353–365. https://doi.org/10.1521/suli.2007.37.3.353

Simon, T. R., Swann, A. C., Powell, K. E., Potter, L. B. Kresnow, M.-J., & O'Carroll, P. W. (2001). Characteristics of impulsive suicide attempts and attempters. *Suicide and Life-Threatening Behavior, 32*(Supplement to Issue 1), 49–59. https://doi.org/10.1521/suli.32.1.5.49.24212

World Health Organization. (2021). *Suicide worldwide in 2019: Global health estimates.* https://www.who.int/publications/i/item/9789240 026643

World Health Organization. (2023). *Suicide.* https://www.who.int/new -room/fact-sheets/detail/suicide

World Health Organization. (2024a). *Suicide prevention.* https://www .who.int/health-topics/suicide#tab=tab_1

World Health Organization. (2024b). *Suicide rates.* https://www.who.int /data/gho/data/themes/mental-health/suicide-rates

SEVENTEEN | Psychotic Episodes

CASSANDRA IS A 24-YEAR-OLD GRADUATE STUDENT *who grew up in a large, close-knit family in a small town on the Eastern Seaboard. She attended a small local college, often returning home for dinners or weekends. Wanting to expand her horizons, she applied to graduate school and was accepted at a large university on the West Coast. This marked the first time she had been away from her hometown and her family for an extended period. While her aunt had been diagnosed with bipolar disorder, Cassandra herself had never experienced any significant psychological problems.*

The transition to graduate school was difficult. Though Cassandra made friends, they were not as supportive as her undergraduate peers. The coursework was also quite challenging. She was averaging four to five hours of sleep per night and often relied on high-potency energy drinks — two or three 16-ounce cans several times a week — to complete assignments. She increased her consumption during midterms.

Cassandra completed her midterms on Thursday and texted her friend Ashley to see if she wanted to go to the movies on Friday night to relax. Ashley agreed to meet Cassandra for the 11 p.m. showing.

Feeling exhausted before the movie, Cassandra had another energy drink, this one containing more caffeine than three cups of regular coffee. The movie they chose to watch was rather cutting edge and required considerable concentration. It was not the "relaxing" experience they had hoped for. After about 30 minutes into the film, just as Ashley was about to suggest they leave, Cassandra began speaking to the characters on-screen in a conversational tone, as if they were addressing her directly. At first, Ashley chuckled. But she soon realized Cassandra was fully engaged, behaving as though she were a character in the film. Cassandra also stood up repeatedly, distracting others from enjoying the movie. Several people told her to sit down and be quiet. Cassandra seemed unaware of them and remained fully immersed in the movie's dialogue. For Cassandra, this was no longer a movie; it had come alive, and she was in it.

Ashley, who had taken several psychology classes as an undergraduate, recognized that Cassandra's behavior seemed consistent with a syndrome she had studied: a brief psychotic episode.

What Is Psychosis?

Psychosis is a combination of signs and symptoms that distort a person's thoughts or perceptions of reality. Its estimated lifetime global prevalence is about 0.8% (Moreno-Küstner et al., 2018), meaning it affects about 64 million people.

Key Features: Signs and Symptoms

In general, psychosis is thought to manifest through "positive" and "negative" symptoms.

Positive Symptoms

The term "positive symptoms" in psychosis can be misleading. Typically, the word "positive" implies something helpful or encouraging. In the context of psychosis, however, this is not the case. Positive symptoms refer to thoughts or behaviors that occur only in those with psychosis—added or "positive" symptoms that are not present in those without the condition. These are essentially new thoughts or behaviors that add to or distort perceptions of reality.

According to the *DSM-5-TR* (American Psychiatric Association [APA], 2022), the positive signs and symptoms of psychosis include the following:

- *Hallucinations*—experiencing sensations that are not real. The most common type is auditory (hearing—e.g., voices, music, television, nature sounds), but there are also visual (seeing—e.g., people, objects, animals, shapes), olfactory (smelling—e.g., something pleasant like baking or something unpleasant like burning rubber), tactile (touch—e.g., bugs, something scratching), and gustatory (taste—e.g., metal, bitterness, sweet, salt) hallucinations.
- *Delusions*—false beliefs that persist despite clear evidence to the contrary. Common types include grandiosity (belief that one has special powers or abilities), persecutory (belief that one is being harassed or targeted, such as being followed or poisoned), referential (belief that comments or signals are directed at them, e.g., the television is talking directly to them), and nihilistic (belief that a tragedy or disaster is imminent).
- *Disorganized speech*—speech that often makes little sense, contains irrational content, jumps from topic to topic, or uses made-up words (known as neologisms).

- *Disorganized or abnormal behavior*—behavior that is impulsive or agitated, interferes with completion of daily tasks, or shows decreased or impaired responsiveness to the environment or environmental cues (catatonia).

Negative Symptoms

Like positive symptoms, the term "negative symptoms" in psychosis can also be misleading. We typically think of "negative" as meaning harmful or destructive. In the context of psychosis, however, negative symptoms refer to deficits—the reduction or absence of certain experiences, such as emotions, behaviors, and normal thought processes—in those with psychosis that are not observed in those without the condition (Lutgens et al., 2017).

Negative symptoms include:

- Reduced personal hygiene
- Decreased interest or pleasure in activities
- Decreased interest in family or friends (social withdrawal)
- Difficulty expressing emotion
- Mood swings or lack of motivation (lethargy)
- Uneasiness around others, interacting awkwardly
- Emotionally flat or minimally responsive
- Low energy
- Reduced speech or difficulty expressing themselves

Types of Psychosis and Psychotic Episodes

There is no single cause of psychosis; it is thought to result from a complex blend of genetics, neurological predispositions, and environmental exposure. Certain combinations of psychotic symptoms occur in recognizable diagnostic patterns (known as psychotic disorders), which are included in the *DSM-5-TR* (APA, 2022). Some of them are described below.

Schizophrenia

Schizophrenia is the most recognized of the psychotic disorders. According to the World Health Organization (WHO, 2022), it affects about 0.32% of the global population (around 26 million people), of whom an estimated 2.22 million are in the United States (National Institute of Mental Health, n.d.). Despite its relatively low prevalence compared to some other disorders like depression (see Chapter Five) and anxiety (see Chapter Eight), schizophrenia places a tremendous health, social, and economic burden on patients and families (Chong et al., 2016). For example, those with schizophrenia live about 15–20 years less than those in the general population, a gap attributed to various factors such as cardiovascular disease, cancer, infections, and lifestyle-related issues such as smoking, substance use, sedentary behavior, and limited access to quality health care (Peritogiannis et al., 2022).

Although quite variable in pattern and course, schizophrenia often begins in young adulthood with a prodromal period—warning signs and symptoms that precede the disorder's onset. This period is characterized by a combination of many negative symptoms, such as deteriorating personal functioning, concentration problems, unusual ideas, apathy, and reduced ability to maintain daily activities. It is typically followed by an acute episode of positive symptoms (e.g., hallucinations, delusions, behavioral disturbances) that cause distress (National Institute for Health and Care Excellence, 2014). A diagnosis is made when psychosis symptoms persist for at least six months, accompanied by marked disruption in functioning (APA, 2022).

Treatments to help resolve positive symptoms typically include medications, which can be very effective, along with psychological therapies and other supportive interventions. For instance, regular physical activity has been shown to be beneficial for many negative symptoms (Swora et al., 2022).

One of the biggest challenges associated with schizophrenia is the considerable stigma surrounding it, along with the public's fear of interacting with those who have the condition. Despite the perception that individuals with schizophrenia are inherently violent, evidence shows they are more likely to be victims of violence than perpetrators (Fitzgerald et al., 2005; Wehring & Carpenter, 2011).

Bipolar Disorder with Psychotic Features

Bipolar disorder (formerly known as manic-depressive disorder) is diagnosed when a person experiences recurring episodes of mania—or a milder form known as hypomania—typically preceded or followed by a depressive episode lasting at least two weeks (see Chapter Five). A manic episode is a distinct period of persistently elevated, irritable, or fluctuating mood that lasts at least seven days and is evident for most of the day. It is accompanied by behaviors such as a decreased need for sleep (sometimes going days without sleeping), racing thoughts, fast or pressured speech, tirades, topic shifts while talking, distractibility, multitasking, and impulsivity often combined with poor decision-making (e.g., spending sprees, driving several hundred miles recklessly). These symptoms impair functioning and are not attributable to a medical condition or substance use (APA, 2022). Bipolar disorder with psychotic features involves delusions and/or hallucinations occurring during a manic or depressive episode.

Depression with Psychotic Features

Depression with psychotic features occurs when delusions and/or hallucinations are present at any time during a depressive episode (see Chapter Five).

Substance-Induced Psychosis

Substance-induced psychosis, also referred to as drug-induced psychosis, is characterized by the presence of delusions and/or hallucinations caused by alcohol or drug use (see Chapter Thirteen). Importantly, these symptoms occur in addition to the expected effects of the substance. They may appear during intoxication, during withdrawal, or, in some instances, may persist after withdrawal (APA, 2022).

Brief Psychotic Episodes

A person can experience psychosis without meeting the criteria for any of the formal diagnoses described above. That is likely the case for Cassandra. An estimated 2–7% of individuals who experience their first episode of psychosis have a brief psychotic episode (Castagnini & Fusar-Poli, 2017), which the DSM-5-TR classifies as brief psychotic disorder (BPD) (APA, 2022). BPD involves the sudden onset of psychotic symptoms — at least one of which must be delusions, hallucinations, or disorganized speech — that last for at least one day but resolve within a month, either on their own or with treatment (e.g., medication), and the person returns to their previous level of functioning.

It is important to recognize that some symptoms of BPD — such as seeing or hearing the deceased, or speaking seemingly incoherently — may occur as part of a ritual or cultural ceremony. In these instances, the experiences should not be classified as symptoms of BPD. In a study from Finland, the prevalence of BPD is estimated to be 0.05% of the general population (Perälä et al., 2007). The chance of recurrence has been reported at approximately 37% over a two-year period (Provenzani et al., 2021).

Relevant to E-PFA, BPD may be triggered by extreme trauma or stress, such as the death of a loved one (see Chapter Fifteen), assault, or a disaster (see Chapter Eleven). This subtype—BPD with an obvious stressor—is also known as brief reactive psychosis (WebMD, 2022). There were anecdotal reports of brief reactive psychosis among first responders in the weeks and months after the terrorist attacks of September 11, 2001. BPD is also observed in individuals experiencing inordinate or chronic stress, such as immigrants, asylum seekers, and refugees (APA, 2022; Brandt et al., 2019).

There has been considerable interest over the past 10 to 15 years in BPD occurring in women during the perinatal period—that is, during pregnancy or more often suddenly postpartum. While postpartum depression was mentioned in Chapter Five, this more severe condition is referred to as postpartum psychosis. Although postpartum BPD typically begins 3 to 10 days after delivery (Friedman et al., 2023), cases have been reported as late as six months after delivery (Monzon et al., 2014). The estimated global prevalence of postpartum BPD is 1 to 2 cases per 1,000 births (Vander-Kruik et al., 2017). Notably, although 40% of women with postpartum psychosis have no prior history of severe mental illness, those with a history of bipolar disorder are at higher risk (Perry et al., 2021).

Underlying Conditions Associated with Psychosis

In addition to formally diagnosed types, psychosis can also result from a variety of medical or physical conditions, according to the Cleveland Clinic (2022), including:

- Dementia
- Dehydration
- Hormonal conditions
- Infections

- Multiple sclerosis
- Lyme disease
- Stroke
- Injury (e.g., head injury)
- Vitamin deficiencies (e.g., B1 or thiamine, B12)

Potential E-PFA Recommendations
(Think About Trying This)

What can Cassandra's friend Ashley do to assist Cassandra with this apparent episode of psychosis? Let's look at the situation through the five-phase E-PFA lens. Listed below are potential E-PFA interventions that might help someone in a situation similar to Cassandra's.

Keep in mind that psychotic reactions — especially those that are brief and seem reactive — may arise from one or more of at least three overarching conditions:

1) Extreme stress or depression (brief reactive psychosis). The combined stress of academic demands and moving across the country may be factors contributing to Cassandra's auditory hallucinations.

2) External physical factors, such as head injury, hallucinogenic drugs, extreme heat, new prescription drug interactions, dehydration, sleep deprivation, certain poisons, and even excessive consumption of popular dietary or energy stimulants. Sleep deprivation and excessive use of energy drinks may have contributed to Cassandra's hallucinations.

3) Diagnosed mental disorders, such as schizophrenia, bipolar disorder, and some forms of depression.

In almost all circumstances, the E-PFA intervention for a psychotic episode will be similar to the acute interventions used for anger, panic, intoxication, and suicidal thoughts (see Chapters Nine, Ten, Thirteen, and Sixteen, respectively). Like intoxication and suicidal thoughts, psychosis should be considered a medical emergency.

1) Introduce yourself (if applicable), offer to help, set expectations, de-escalate (if needed).
2) Gather information. (*What happened? What hurts? How bad is it?*) Determine the severity and urgency of the situation.
3) Clarify. Make sure Cassandra's reaction is indeed an alteration in her understanding of reality.
4) Provide assistance. The goals are ensuring safety and accessing professional care.
5) Make a plan. Identify the next steps in securing further care.

Introduce Yourself, Offer to Help, Set Expectations

- E-PFA begins with "showing up," expressing calm, nonconfrontational concern, and helping to de-escalate the situation by getting Cassandra out of the movie theater. Ashley can then reassure Cassandra that she wants to help. Although it may sound unnecessary, Ashley should ensure that Cassandra recognizes her.
- In the case of psychotic experiences, it's imperative to remember that the person is experiencing an alternative reality. Right now, Cassandra's reality is not the same as Ashley's reality. So Cassandra may not perceive herself as being in distress. In some instances, the psychotic experience is perceived as positive or euphoric. With this in mind, the physical safety of both Cassandra and Ashley becomes paramount.

Gather Information

- Ashley should encourage Cassandra to talk about what she is experiencing. Questions like "What's going on?" are a good beginning. She should listen for signs of a psychotic episode, keeping in mind that Cassandra may perceive her experiences as negative and disconcerting, neutral, or even positive. She should gently ask Cassandra for specifics about what she is experiencing. Signs of a possible psychotic episode include the following:

- Hearing voices (as in Cassandra's case)
- Seeing people, places, or things (it's unclear whether Cassandra is experiencing visual hallucinations)
- Smelling unusual odors (olfactory hallucinations)
- Feeling physical sensations, like being touched (tactile hallucinations)
- Experiencing unusual tastes (gustatory hallucinations)
- Out-of-body sensations
- Delusions, most commonly paranoid delusions (irrational suspicions or beliefs)
- Delusions accompanied by voices telling the person to take certain actions (command hallucinations)

- Command hallucinations are often the most concerning type of psychotic reaction. It's important for Ashley to ask Cassandra precisely what the voices are saying, as this can help assess the level of immediate risk to both Cassandra and Ashley.

- Once Cassandra describes her reactions, Ashley may ask, "When did these reactions (i.e., conversations) begin?" She should try to determine whether the reactions are part of a chronic psychological disorder or a situational response to extreme stress, recreational drugs, head injury, sleep deprivation, or some other physical stimulus. In Cassandra's case, the hallucinations seem to be a recent development.

Clarify

- The clarification phase usually begins with a paraphrase or recap of what Ashley has seen and heard from Cassandra. For example, "So, you're saying there are voices that are speaking directly to you?"
- If Cassandra asks whether Ashley hears the voices, Ashley should be honest. She might say something like, "I don't hear the voices the way you seem to be hearing them, but if you say you are having a conversation with them, I believe you."

Provide Assistance

Problem-Focused

- In this context, it is most reasonable to identify the problem as the psychotic auditory (and possibly visual) hallucinations Cassandra is experiencing. Therefore, Ashley's first priority should be ensuring mutual safety. It is also important for her to consider and rule out other potential causes, such as a medical issue or the influences of substances (drugs or medications).
- Next, Ashley should consider the psychotic reaction, along with its potential behavioral correlates and consequences, as a medical emergency.

Emotion-Focused

- Emotion-focused E-PFA during Cassandra's apparent psychotic episode would consist of Ashley avoiding argumentation, confrontation, or any other action that might provoke an escalation.
- Consistent with that, Ashley can encourage a discussion of topics that are likely to be calming or even positively distracting.
- In Cassandra's case, Ashley might ask her to describe the conversation in detail, as long as doing so does not increase Cassandra's distress. The goal is not to reinforce the psychotic reaction but to

de-escalate the situation, show Cassandra that Ashley is trying to understand rather than argue, and prepare for the transition to professional care.

Stress Management-Focused

- Stress management-focused intervention involves acute de-escalation techniques, discussed in previous chapters, or even introducing methods like thought substitution (replacing unwanted thoughts with more adaptive or positive ones) or thought stopping (interrupting and halting unwanted thoughts to prevent escalation). Cassandra may feel an overwhelming loss of personal control, which can fuel the psychotic process. Any techniques Ashley can employ to help Cassandra regain a sense of control will be useful during the transition to professional care.

Make a Plan

- As mentioned, a brief psychotic episode should be considered a medical emergency. Ashley should respond accordingly by calling 9-1-1 or seeking emergency medical support through other available means.
- When possible, it is best to obtain the cooperation of the person in crisis, and to seek assistance from friends or family members who can provide a calming and supportive presence. In Cassandra's case, eliciting the help of family members is unlikely, so Ashley will need to act with some urgency.
- While avoiding argumentation as much as possible, Ashley might say to Cassandra, "Sounds like we have an issue that we need help with. You are telling me the actors in the movie were carrying on a conversation with you, actually responding to what you were saying. But no one else around you heard the voices in the same way. In fact, many people were asking you to be quiet and sit down. Neither of us can explain what's going on, so I think

it's important that we get some help. What you are going through seems pretty confusing. Let's see what we can do to figure this out. And the best way to start is to call 9-1-1."

E-PFA Dialogue (It Might Sound Like This)

ASHLEY (QUIETLY): Cassandra, can you hear me?

CASSANDRA (NOT LOOKING AT ASHLEY): Huh, what?

ASHLEY: Cassandra, it's me Ashley. I'm sitting next to you.

CASSANDRA (LOOKING OVER AND RECOGNIZING ASHLEY): Ashley?

ASHLEY: Yes, it's me. Will you walk outside with me? I want to try and help you.

CASSANDRA: But I'm in the middle of an interesting conversation that I want to finish. I don't need any help right now.

ASHLEY (CALMLY): I hear that's what you want to do, but I would really appreciate it if you would take a walk with me.

CASSANDRA (PAUSING): Okay, but this better be important. (*Addressing the screen.*) Excuse me, I'll be right back.

(*Cassandra follows Ashley outside. The two sit down on a bench near the street.*)

ASHLEY: Thanks for walking outside and sitting with me, Cassandra. I want to make sure we're okay—that we're safe.

CASSANDRA: Safe? Why wouldn't we be safe? I feel perfectly safe. In fact, I feel great.

ASHLEY: Tell me what's going on?

CASSANDRA: I just met those interesting people inside and was part of a really inspiring conversation. It was kind of difficult to follow, so I'd really like to get back to it.

ASHLEY: What was the conversation about?

CASSANDRA: We were talking about lying to ourselves, and how reflections in mirrors often create a desire to dance with shadows. And how these shadows dampen our dreams, but in our search, we create constellations of hope.

ASHLEY: Hmmm . . . that's kind of hard for me to understand. What do you make of it? Do you think there's anything risky in what they're saying?

CASSANDRA: Oh gosh, no. I was thrilled to be part of it.

ASHLEY: When did this conversation begin?

CASSANDRA: Less than 10 minutes ago, when I was invited into it.

ASHLEY: So, you're saying there are voices speaking directly to you?

CASSANDRA: Yes, weren't they speaking directly to you?

ASHLEY: I didn't hear the voices the way you seem to be hearing them, but if you say you are having a conversation with them, I believe you.

CASSANDRA: What are you saying, Ashley? They weren't talking to you? I'm sorry you weren't part of the conversation. But wait a minute . . . is something wrong? Are we okay?

ASHLEY: I am here with you, and I'm going to help make sure that everything is going to be okay. Besides the conversation you're a part of, are you seeing, smelling, or feeling anything else that you want to tell me about?

CASSANDRA: Well, I saw the people in the theater, but mostly heard the conversations. I don't think there's anything else to tell you about. What's going on?

ASHLEY: I'm not sure, but I want to help. Do you mind if I ask you something else?

CASSANDRA: You can ask me whatever you want, Ashley.

ASHLEY: I'm not trying to pry, but have you taken any medications or any other substances that might be harmful?

CASSANDRA: No! Why would you ask that? I mean, I haven't been sleeping well for the past month, and that got worse as I was going through midterms. Thank goodness my exams ended yesterday. The only thing that I've been doing more of is drinking energy drinks. I'll admit that. In fact, I had a new one right before I left to meet you tonight because I was tired. The label said that it's got the caffeine content of three cups of coffee, as well as taurine and guarana.

ASHLEY: Thanks for sharing that, Cassandra. That's helpful to know. Anything else—like any medical issues? For you or your family?

CASSANDRA: Not for me . . . or my parents. I don't know if this means anything, but my aunt has bipolar disorder, and there are times when she's acted erratically. Why are you asking?

ASHLEY: I'm just trying to get some information. (*Redirecting Cassandra to avoid escalation.*) Listen, before we talk more about the conversation you were having inside, I want to hear more about the vacation you said you're planning for the summer.

CASSANDRA: Oh, that's right. I can't wait. I'm heading to Aruba, 10 days, all included. The offer still stands for you to join me.

ASHLEY: It's really tempting. I'll have to see if I can get away. Either way, it sounds like a wonderful time for you.

CASSANDRA: I wonder if anyone I just met inside would be interested in going. I'm always up for others joining me for an adventure. And besides, they seem so interesting based on our conversation, although it was a little overwhelming.

ASHLEY: Any more information you'd like to share with me about the conversation you had with them?

CASSANDRA: Hmmm . . . I wasn't aware of this before, but I can still hear the conversation now even though I don't see them. They're talking about how we need to carve out our destinies by making good choices, and they're asking for my input. There's more than one voice, and they're all talking at once. It's interesting, but they're not stopping, and sometimes they're getting louder. Ashley, I'm starting to feel like I'm losing control.

ASHLEY: I hear what you're saying. Is it okay if I hold your hand?

CASSANDRA: Yes . . . please.

ASHLEY (TAKING CASSANDRA'S HAND): Let's try a few things to help you feel a little more in control right now. We could talk about something pleasant, like your vacation. You can remind yourself that I'm here with you and it's safe. You can ask the voices to stop or imagine putting a stop sign in front of them. Or we could do that breathing exercise from the yoga class we took six months ago.

CASSANDRA (VOICE SHAKY): What's going on, Ashley?

ASHLEY (CALMLY): It's going to be okay, but we have an issue that we need help with. You said the actors in the movie are talking with you, actually responding to what you're saying.

But no one else seemed to hear them the same way. People around us were asking you to be quiet and sit down. Neither of us can explain what's going on, so I think it's important that we get some help. What you're going through seems very confusing. Let's see what we can do to figure this out. The best way to do that is to call 9-1-1. I'm going to make that call, and while we wait, let's do the breathing technique together and keep talking until they arrive. I'm right here with you.

CASSANDRA: Okay.

References

American Psychiatric Association. (2022). Schizophrenia spectrum and other psychotic disorders. In *Diagnostic and statistical manual of mental disorders* (5th ed., text rev.). https://doi.org/10.1176/appi.books.9780890425787.x02_Schizophrenia_Spectrum

Brandt, L., Henssler, J., Müller, M., Wall, S., Gabel, D., & Heinz, A. (2019). Risk of psychosis among refugees. *JAMA Psychiatry, 76*(11), 1133–1140. https://doi.org/10.1001/jamapsychiatry.2019.1937

Castagnini, A. C., & Fusar-Poli, P. (2017). Diagnostic validity of ICD-10 acute and transient psychotic disorders and DSM-5 brief psychotic disorder. *European Psychiatry, 45*, 104–113. https://doi.org/10.1016/j.eurpsy.2017.05.028

Chong, H. Y., Teoh, S. L., Wu, D. B., Kotirum, S., Chiou, C., & Chai-yakunapruk, N. (2016). Global economic burden of schizophrenia: A systematic review. *Neuropsychiatric Disease and Treatment, 12*, 357–373. https://doi.org/10.2147/NDT.S96649

Cleveland Clinic. (2022). *Overview: What is psychosis?* https://my.clevelandclinic.org/health/symptoms/23012-psychosis

Fitzgerald, P. B., De Castella, A. R., Filia, K. M., Filia, S. L., Benitez, J., & Kulkarni, J. (2005). Victimization of patients with schizophrenia and related disorders. *Australian and New Zealand Journal of Psychiatry, 39*(3), 169–174. https://doi.org/10.1080/j.1440-1614.2005.01539.x

Friedman, S. H., Reed, E., & Ross, N. E. (2023). Postpartum psychosis. *Current Psychiatry Reports, 25,* 65–72. https://doi.org/10.1007/s11920 -022-01406-4

Lutgens, D., Gariepy, G., & Malla, A. (2017). Psychological and psycho- social interventions for negative symptoms in psychosis: Systematic review and meta-analysis. *The British Journal of Psychiatry, 210*(5), 324–332. https://doi.org/10.1192/bjp.bp.116.197103

Monzon, C., di Scalea, T. L., & Pearlstein, T. (2014). Postpartum psychosis: Updates and clinical issues. *Psychiatric Times, 31*(1), 1-6.

Moreno-Küstner, B., Martin, C., & Pastor, L. (2018). Prevalence of psychotic disorders and its association with methodological issues. A systematic review and meta-analyses. *PLOS One.* https://doi.org .10.1371/journal.pone.0195687

National Institute for Health and Care Excellence. (2014). *Psychosis and schizophrenia in adults: Prevention and management.* https://www.nice .org.uk/guidance/CG178/chapter/introduction

National Institute of Mental Health (NIMH). (n.d.). *Schizophrenia.* https://www.nimh.nih.gov/health/statistics/schizophrenia

Perälä, J., Suvisaari, J., Saarni, S. I., Kuoppalasmi, K., Isometsä, E., Pirkola, S., Partonen, T., Tuulio-Henriksson, A., Hintikka, J., Kieseppä, T., Härkänen, T., Koskinen, S., & Lönnqvist, J. (2007). Lifetime prevalence of psychotic and bipolar I disorders in a general population. *Archives of General Psychiatry, 64*(1), 19–28. https://doi.org/10.1001/archpsyc.64.1.19

Peritogiannis, V., Ninou, A., & Samakouri, M. (2022). Mortality in schizophrenia-spectrum disorders: Recent advances in understand- ing and management. *Healthcare, 10*(12). https://doi.org/10.3390/health care10122366

Perry, A., Gordon-Smith, K., Di Florio, A., Craddock, N., Jones, L., & Jones, I. (2021). Mood episodes in pregnancy and risk of postpartum recurrence in bipolar disorder: The Bipolar Disorder Research Network Pregnancy Study. *Journal of Affective Disorders, 294,* 714–722. https://doi.org/10.1016/j.jad.2021.07.067

Provenzani, U., Salazar de Pablo, G., Arribas, M., Pillman, F., & Fusar-Poli, P. (2021). Clinical outcomes in brief psychotic episodes: A systematic review and meta-analysis. *Epidemiology and Psychiatric Sciences, 30,* e71, 1-10. https://doi.org/10.1017/S2045796021000548

Swora, E., Boberska, M., Kulis, E., Knoll, N., Keller, J., & Luszczynska, A. (2022). Physical activity, positive and negative symptoms of psychosis, and general psychopathology among people with psychotic disorders: A meta-analysis. *Journal of Clinical Medicine, 11*(10), 2719. https://doi.org/10.3390/jcm11102719

VanderKruik, R., Barreix, M., Chou, D., Allen, T., Say, L., Cohen, L. S., on behalf of the Maternal Morbidity Working Group. (2017). The global prevalence of postpartum psychosis: A systematic review. *BMC Psychiatry, 17* (272). https/doi.org/10.1186/s12888-017-1427-7

WebMD. (2022). *What is brief psychotic disorder?* https://www.webmd .com/schizophrenia/mental-health-brief-pscyhotic-disorder

Wehring, H. J., & Carpenter, W. T. (2011). Violence and schizophrenia. *Schizophrenia Bulletin, 37*(5), 877–878. https://doi.org/10.1093/schbul /sbr094

World Health Organization. (2022). *Schizophrenia.* https://www.who .int/news-room/fact-sheets/detail/schizophrenia

ACKNOWLEDGMENTS

TO O. LEE MCCABE, PHD AND BERTRAM BROWN, MD, MPH
you both have taught me much about crisis and life.

To Patti Copps for your love and support as this book was written.

And let us not forget Sir Winston Churchill, who reminds us that to each of us there comes a special moment when we are offered a chance to do something special, perhaps helping another who is in acute distress. This book will help us all prepare for that moment—a moment that could be our finest hour. (GSE)

This project—to make our work in psychological first aid widely accessible—represents the culmination of decades of academic and applied experience. I would like to express my sincere gratitude to the following individuals for their invaluable contributions, both direct and indirect.

I extend my heartfelt thanks to Stephen F. Bono, PhD, for his nearly thirty-five years of mentorship and friendship. In recent years, I have been fortunate to receive guidance, support, and develop a deeper friendship with Eric Lane, PsyD, and Melissa Lane,

MA. I also want to acknowledge Mark Danzig, from the US Department of State, Claudine Meyer-Sager, MS, Head of CISM from the Swiss Air Navigation Services, Allan McDougall, founder of the All Labor Movement (ALM), Duronda Pope, Director of the Emergency Response Team (ERT) of the United Steelworkers (USW), Mendy Coën, Director General of the United States Chaplain Corps (USCC), and Staff Sergeant Ray Savage, developer of the National Reintegration Program (NRP) from the Royal Canadian Mounted Police (RCMP), for their continued inspiration, passion, and persistence over many years in advancing the application of peer support, psychological first aid, and crisis intervention in their respective fields. I am truly grateful to be part of your remarkable communities.

I also wish to thank my exceptional colleagues at Loyola University Maryland, especially my next-door office neighbor and friend, Matthew Kirkhart, PhD.

Most importantly, I am forever grateful to my family for their unwavering grounding, comfort, support, humor, and providing a place to call home. (JML)

We wish to thank O. Lee McCabe, PhD, retired faculty member of the Johns Hopkins School of Medicine and the Johns Hopkins Bloomberg School of Public Health, who has made significant scientific contributions to the field of disaster preparedness and psychological first aid. Dr. McCabe is also the namesake of the McCabe Professorship in the Neuropsychopharmacology of Consciousness, an endowed position in the Johns Hopkins Department of Psychiatry and Behavioral Sciences. His professional and personal influence continues to be a profound source of inspiration for us. A special acknowledgment and thanks to Amelie Burns for her organizational and editorial assistance, and thanks to Emma Ginn Wilkie for her help reviewing references.

Finally, we extend our gratitude to Robin W. Coleman, Marlee Brooks, Jennifer D'Urso, Kristina Lykke, and Edith Saint Preux, from Johns Hopkins University Press, and to project editor Mary C. Ribesky and copyeditor Kelley Blewster, for their willingness to push for adoption of this unique text, their patience throughout the project, and their editorial and marketing assistance. (GSE and JML)

INDEX

33–34; for depression, 74–78; for eating disorder, 197–200; for fear, 121–23; for grief, 265–68; for guilt, 251–54; for intoxication, 209–14; for panic attacks/disorder, 164–67; for psychosis/psychotic episodes, 299–303; for stress, 97–100; for suicidal thoughts, 280–85; tailoring to each unique situation, 2, 29; for traumatic stress, 179–83. *See also* dialogue, E-PFA

intoxicants: alcohol, 218–22; cannabis (marijuana), 222–24; cocaine, 224–27; effects of, 208–9; ketamine, 236–39; MDMA (Ecstasy), 230–33; multiple use of, 240; opioids, 227–30; psilocybin, 233–36; reasons for using, 207

intoxication: definition, 207; dialogue with someone experiencing, 214–17; intervention for, 209–14; physical symptoms of, 209; psychological symptoms of, 208–9; scenario involving, 206–7; severity of, 207

introducing yourself, in E-PFA model, 16, 24, 25, 28, 30, 31–32; to person experiencing panic, 164–65; to someone experiencing traumatic stress, 180; for traumatic events, 179–80. *See also* de-escalation; help, offering; "showing up"

introspection, solving or mitigating problems through, 39, 40

Johns Hopkins Center for Public Health Preparedness, 12–13, 21

Johns Hopkins Guide to Psychological First Aid, The, 2, 14–15

Johns Hopkins Model of Everyday Psychological First Aid (E-PFA), 14–17. *See also* E-PFA (everyday psychological first aid)

Johns Hopkins University School of Medicine, 236

journaling, 47

Journal of Clinical Psychology, 20

Jung, Carl, 40

ketamine, 236–39

Kübler-Ross, Elisabeth, 260

Law of Effect, 40

laws of operant conditioning, 40

legalization, of marijuana, 224

LGBTI population, 193, 276

life-threatening impairment, blood alcohol content (BAC) levels, 222

limbic system, 111, 208

Lindemann, Erich, 260

listening, reflective, 60–61

loneliness, 9–10, 262

LSD (lysergic acid diethylamide), 232, 236

Lyme disease, 299

"magic mushrooms," 234

major depression, 73, 236

marijuana (cannabis), 222–24

McGregor, Douglas, 14

MDMA (Ecstasy), 230–33, 237

medical emergencies: for eating disorder, 199, 200; for intoxication, 211, 217, 218; for panic, 166; for psychotic episode, 300–302; for suicidal thoughts, 280. *See also* 9-1-1, calling

medical marijuana, 224

medications, 47, 166, 211

meditation, 47, 100, 182

Merck Pharmaceuticals, 232

mescaline, 236

methadone, 228

migraines, 96, 152, 222

mild depression, 71

About the Authors

George S. Everly, Jr., PhD, MA, ABPP, FACLP, is considered one of the world's leading authorities on psychological crisis intervention and one of the founding fathers of the field of disaster mental health. He is a public health scholar and clinical psychologist and has held faculty appointments at the Johns Hopkins Bloomberg School of Public Health, the Johns Hopkins School of Medicine, and Harvard University, among other institutions. He was formerly Chief Psychologist and Director of Behavioral Medicine at the Johns Hopkins Homewood Hospital Center, and the founding chairperson for Central Maryland's branch of the American Red Cross disaster mental health team. In addition, he served the Office of His Highness the Amir of Kuwait after the first Gulf War, the New York Police Department after the World Trade Center disaster of September 11, 2001, the Department of Homeland Security's Infrastructure Protection Team, the FBI National Academy, the Bureau of Alcohol, Tobacco, Firearms and Explosives (ATF) Peer Support Team, the Hospital Authority of Hong Kong after the SARS pandemic, and the Johns Hopkins Medical Institutions during and after the COVID-19 pandemic. Dr. Everly is author and coauthor of more than twenty books, including the national bestseller *Lodestar*. He has been invited to lecture in over thirty countries on six continents. From 1990 to mid-2025, Dr. Everly was the top ranked author in the world on the topic of psychological first aid, according to *PubMed PubReMiner*.

Jeffrey M. Lating, PhD, earned his BA in psychology from Swarthmore College and his PhD in clinical psychology from the University of Georgia. He completed a postdoctoral fellowship in medical psychology at Johns Hopkins Hospital. He is currently a professor of psychology at Loyola University Maryland, where he received the 2025 Harry W. Rodgers III Distinguished Teacher of the Year award. Dr. Lating has coedited and coauthored seven books on stress, posttraumatic stress, and psychological first aid. As a consultant and trainer, he has worked with the Federal Emergency Management Agency (FEMA), the Bureau of Alcohol, Tobacco, Firearms and Explosives (ATF), and the US Senate Employee Assistance Program (EAP). In addition, his contributions have supported the Association of Professional Flight Attendants (APFA), the United Steelworkers (USW), and the National Association of Letter Carriers (NALC), as well as international organizations including the Danish Military, the Royal Canadian Mounted Police (RCMP), the Swiss Air Navigation Services, and the World Bank. Notably, he provided interventions with the US Secret Service's EAP in New York City following the September 11, 2001, terrorist attacks.

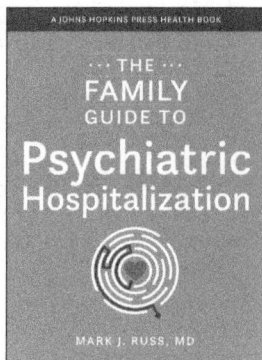

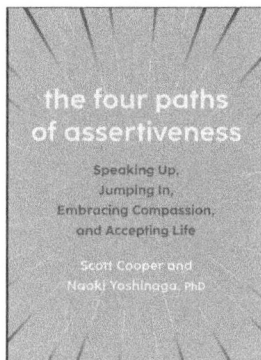

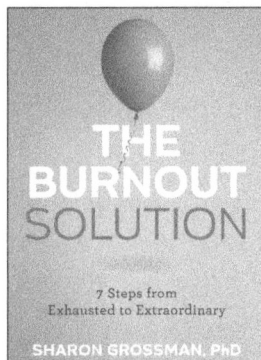

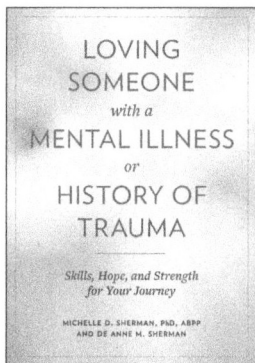

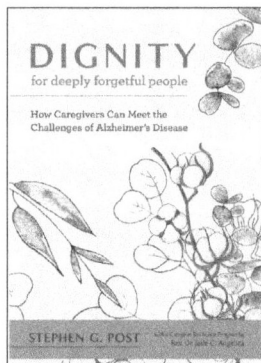

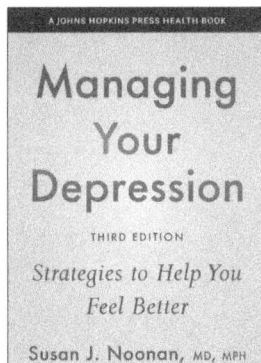